The mR40 Method

The 40 Day Guide to Reset Your Metabolism, Lose Weight and Optimize Your Health

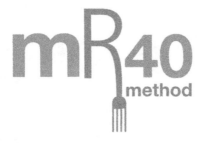

By Mubarakah Ibrahim

Disclaimer & Copyright

The author, publisher, and distributors of this book are not responsible for any consequences regarding the procedures and suggestions given in this book.

This book is not intended as medical or health advice. We recommend consulting with a health professional before changing your diet or starting an exercise program.

Apart from personal use, no part of this publication may be reproduced or distributed, in any form or by any means; electronic, mechanical, photocopying, or otherwise, without prior written permission from the publisher.

If you like and/or feel benefitted by the information in this program, we would encourage you to show your support by sharing your testimonial with us, sharing with your friends and family.

First published by Dog Ear Publishing
8888 Keystone Crossing
Suite 1300
Indianapolis, IN 46240
www.dogearpublishing.net

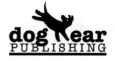

ISBN: 978-145757-077-3

This book is printed on acid-free paper.
Printed in the United States of America

Table of Contents

Preface ix

Introduction xiii

"Unlearn What I Have Learned".. xiii

Welcome to Your 40-Day Metabolic Reset! xix

Chapter 1: What is the mR40 Method... 1

What Makes the mR40 Method Different from Other Keto Programs?....... 3

What Makes the mR40 Method Different from Atkins?................ 3

Why 40 Days and Not 21 Days?.. 4

The 40-Day Transformations 5

Chapter 2: Eat, Stop, Eat: Intermittent Fasting 7

A Historical View of Fasting 9

What Is Intermittent Fasting and How Is It Different from Starving?........ 10

How Does Intermittent Fasting Help with Weight Loss? 11

Stop Starving: Ghrelin and Leptin 12

Fat Loss by Any Other Name: Lipolysis.................................... 14

Muscle Is As Muscle Does 15

Anti-Inflammatory: Human Growth Hormone.......................... 16

What Is Inflammation? 16

Intermittent Fasting Terms.. 18

mR40 Intermittent Fasting 19

Jump-start 19

Phase I 20

Phase II 20

Chapter 3: Key To What? Ketosis Explained 22

What Is Ketosis? 23

How Does a Ketogenic Diet Actually Work? 24

How Does Ketosis Help You Lose Weight? 25

The Domino Effect: Insulin 26

Health Effects of Ketosis That Will Change Your Life 27

Cellular Detox: Autophagy 28

Brain Boost. Mental Focus and Clarity 29

Fountain of Youth? 32

Keto Terms 33

Chapter 4: Got Fat? 35

What Is Ketogenic Eating and Why Do You Want to Do It? 36

Where Did the Ketogenic Diet Come From? 38

A Brief Historical Snapshot of the Use of Ketogenic Eating 39

The Evolution of the Keto Diet 40

Keto Nutrition 41

Macro and Micronutrients 44

Ketogenic Macronutrient Ratio 48

Carb Tracking on a Ketogenic Plan 49

How to Tell If You Are in Ketosis 51

Physical Signs of Ketosis…or at least getting there 51

How to Measure Ketones 52

What Is the Keto Flu? 55

How to minimize the symptoms and duration of the keto flu ... 55

Is the keto flu the same as ketoacidosis? 57

Chapter 5: Fat Guards - Angiogenesis-Inhibiting Foods 58

The Health Affect? 60

AI Fat Guards? 61

AI Foods and Their Benefits 62

Chapter 6: Move … Faster **66**

Get HIIT 70

    mR40 Method Workouts 72

    How to Do mR40 HIIT Training 74

Hack Your Workout Results 77

    Multi-muscle movements 77

Chapter 7: Putting It All Together **79**

Goal Setting 80

    Define Your Goals, Motivation, and Commitment (Find Your Why) 81

    Further Goal-Setting Tips 81

Do It the WRITE Way 82

    Tracking Your Success 83

Get Naked 83

Chapter 8: Lets Eat…NOT That! **88**

Phase I 89

    Intermittent fasting 89

    What to Eat 89

    What NOT to Eat 92

    Jump Start Your First Week 94

Phase II 99

    Intermittent fasting 100

    Nutrition 100

    What Is Glycemic Load (GL)? 102

    The method behind the madness 103

    Foods in Phase II 103

Chapter 9: Keto Missteps and Pitfalls **106**

Eating Too Much Protein 107

Snacking Too Often 107

Eating "Low-Carb" Processed Foods 107

Chapter 10: Hack Your Weight Loss Results **109**

Water Ways 110

Sleep Away the Fat 113

Big Fat Worry Warts: Stress = Fat 118

Chapter 11: But Wait...I Have Some Questions 127

Keto FAQ 128

AI Foods FAQ 129

Intermittent Fasting FAQ 130

mR40 method FAQ 130

Chapter 12: Seven-Day Meal Plan 133

Chapter 13: Food and Recipes 138

Hot Beverages 139

    mR40 Keto Coffee 139

    mR40 Keto Chai 139

Breakfast Options 140

    Loaded Veggie Omelet 140

    Keto Hash Brown 141

    Breakfast Turkey Patties 142

Lunch / Dinner 143

    Spinach Mozzarella Stuffed Burgers 143

    Keto Fried Chicken 144

    Bok Choy Stir Fry with Ground Turkey 145

    Crispy Curry Rubbed Chicken Thigh 146

    Seared Salmon with Sautéed Spinach and Mushrooms ... 147

    Ground Turkey, Ginger, and Garlic Bok Choy Stir-Fry ... 148

    Caveman Chili 149

    Garlic Butter Steelhead Trout 150

    Vegetarian Keto Lasagna 151

Sides 153

    Cauliflower Mashed "Potatoes" 153

    Yellow "Rice" 154

Cauliflower Mac n Cheese 155

"Breads" 156

    Keto Buns 156

    Keto Flat Bread (Naan) 157

    Keto Cornbread 158

Keto Snack Ideas 159

Comprehensive mR40 Food List 161

Summary 164

Preface

When I was seven years old, my mother got married and pregnant with my younger sister. I don't remember much from that year other than the fact that after basking in the glory of being the "baby" of five siblings, I now had to be a big sister, and my mother got sick with something called diabetes. I didn't know what it was at the time; all I knew was that if she didn't give herself injections, she would be sick. My mother had gestational diabetes, and after giving birth to my little sister, she was one of roughly half the women who've had gestational diabetes during pregnancy who go on to develop full-fledged Type 2 diabetes after their child's birth.

I learned to drive at thirteen years old. It was not legal, but my mother told me it was a precaution. You see, sometimes she didn't "feel good," and if I ever had to take her to the hospital, she wanted me to be able to drive. Unlike other teenagers who learned to drive because they wanted the responsibility and freedom, I learned to drive because it could mean life or death for my mother.

When I was fourteen years old, we went shopping for clothes before school began. Being an annual event to get the nicest newest outfit, the latest shoes, and the only name-brand clothes I'd probably be able to get all year, it was a big deal. But by the time we got to the second store, my mother started walking slower. She would sit to rest on whatever surface she could find to hold her light five-foot 125-pound frame: the windowsill or the platform the mannequin stood on.

I found the cutest jacket: a jean jacket with rhinestones. I remember because the rapping duo Salt-N-Pepa was popular and I wanted to look and dress like them. But when I brought the jacket over to my mom, she looked out of it. I asked her if she was okay. She responded, "No, I left the house without my insulin and everything looks blurry. I can't see. We have to go home, and you have to drive because I can't see." I left the jacket on the rack next to me, my mom took my arm, and I led her to the car. I drove home that day, at fourteen years old. I was instructed to take a route that put us in close proximity to the hospital just in case my mom passed out. I drove home slowly, but not too slow so I wouldn't draw suspicion from passing police cars. I drove fast but not too fast. Fast enough to get there quickly but not too fast so I wouldn't get pulled over.

At that age I didn't understand how a person gets diabetes, but I knew I hated the disease. I knew I never wanted to get diabetes. Like many African-American folktales, diabetes, referred to as "sugar" by the older generations, is thought to be genetic. An unavoidable part of being black, of growing older, almost a rite of passage. You're older, you get wiser, you get grays, and you "sugar." Getting your "sugar needles" from the doctor was just an indication of age, sort of how you turn forty and have to start getting mammograms.

No matter how many times I heard how my grandmother had diabetes and my mother had diabetes so I—or one of my siblings—was going to get it, I refused to believe it was my fate. Health issues in my family were often a source of discussion. Not how we could avoid them but rather how we were all playing a game of Russian roulette with diabetes and high blood pressure. Discussing who's going to inherit the one thing we knew for sure my mother would leave as an inheritance. We were ignorant to the fact that we could refuse the estate tax that came along with having our mother's nose or her well-shaped legs that seemed to always be toned no matter how much weight she lost or gained, or her smooth, blemish-free skin from head to toe. With her features and assets came the tax of all her health problems.

Twenty-five years later after I made a career of getting other women healthy, my mother called me, as she did periodically, to get health advice that I was pretty sure she wasn't going to follow. She asked, "My doctor referred me to a nutritionist. Do you think I should go?"

"You've had diabetes for twenty-five years, and no one has ever referred you to a nutritionist?" I asked.

"No," she responded in an almost confused tone as if she questioned why I would even assume someone had.

That moment hit me like a lightning bolt, both illuminating the years of health struggles she faced and showing me the painful reality of simply not knowing how to take care of herself. The lack of health knowledge was literally killing her.

All the times we would get upset with her because we thought she intentionally was not taking care of her health. All the times she scoffed, "Just hand me that Pepsi; everything makes my sugar go up." When she self-diagnosed her out-of-control insulin levels and adjusted her own medication. It was not stubbornness but ignorance in the simplest definition of the words "not knowing." All these years she was never taught what having diabetes meant, how food, movement, and stress affect one's health when one has little to no pancreas function.

The doctor who wrote her a letter to say she could no longer be her health-care provider because of her non-compliance failed to educate her beyond a fifteen-minute appointment and admonishment of drinking soda.

This book is dedicated to my mother and all the women who simply need to know how food and movement affect their health. To the women who long to be empowered by knowledge and know how to take agency over their own well-being.

I pray you be granted a long, healthy life full of vibrancy and pure joy.

Introduction

"Unlearn What I Have Learned"

I'm a personal trainer, fitness expert and weight loss coach with 20 years of experience. This is what I do. So, I've helped thousands of women lose weight and regain their health and confidence. At the same time, one would think I'm not supposed to struggle with my weight but life had other plans.

In 2015, life threw me several curve balls. For instance, during an OBGYN appointment, my doctor discovered a growth in my uterus that needed to be removed and tested for cancer. During the two weeks between having the procedure to remove the growth and waiting for the results, I began to reevaluate my entire life.

Despite having a successful business and other significant career milestones like being featured on the Oprah Winfrey Show and being invited to dinner with President Barack Obama for my contribution to health and wellness in America, I was also concerned about all the goals I had not accomplished. I realized these goals had been delayed for far too long.

After receiving the news that the growth was not cancer, I was able to sigh a breath of relief. In addition, this "clean bill of health" provided me with the motivation to make the appropriate adjustments in my life. So, as I mentioned earlier, I knew I needed to begin accomplishing goals - not simply creating a goal but following through and accomplishing goals. And, the first goal on my list was to return to college and graduate. In order to do this, I closed my fitness studio and returned to school full time. Wow! This was definitely a course correction and major life change for me. It was a huge change for my family as well.

In the midst of this huge life change, one of my children unexpectedly began to struggle with mental health issues. They experienced several hospital stays and participated in intensive out-patient treatment plans. Everything seemed to be spiraling out of control. Regularly, I woke up in the middle of the night just looking at the ceiling and worrying. I also remember, during my studies, leaving class to cry in the bathroom. I couldn't figure out how I would have enough time to meet the deadline for my research paper while regularly meeting with mental health professionals and taking my child to her therapist.

During this stressful period of my life, I found comfort in taking car rides alone. Often, I would end up at the ice cream shop. Each time, I told myself I would get a small ice cream cone and the healthy dinner I was going to eat later would balance everything.

I justified my feelings and my weight gain with, *"I'm getting older, I'm supposed to gain weight"*. Or, I would tell myself, "Well, I have hips and a butt now and this is what a real woman is supposed to look like". Honestly, I did not feel comfortable in my own skin. Those were just words I told myself to cope with the fact that I was not ready to make any changes to my eating habits.

At the same time, I realized I was using my hijab (Islamic concept of modest clothing/accessories) as a cover instead of a covering. Meaning, I questioned whether I chose extra loose shirts as a form of modesty or just to cover the rolls of fat I felt so uncomfortable having around my waist. I wondered if I was wearing long shirts to hide my hips because I was being modest or because I was embarrassed by my weight gain. All the time, I knew the truth. I desperately wanted to lose weight. No...I desperately NEEDED to lose weight. As my clothing options dwindled because many items in my closet no longer covered my unwanted belly roles or widening hips, the scale also tipped at

178lbs and I was devastated. With the exceptions of pregnancies, this was the heaviest I had ever been.

Once my child's mental health was stable and I graduated, I set out on a mission to lose the weight I had gained. I resumed my morning runs and got a gym membership so I could do more strength training. I also enrolled in a boot camp and I even hired a personal trainer to give me that extra push. I was working out six days a week including running or hiking 5-10 miles on weekends. I became physically fit AND absolutely exhausted.

I stopped soothing myself with ice cream and junk food and began to choose healthier food options. For breakfast, I had fruit and veggie smoothies. Throughout the day, I ate low fat foods, lots of veggies and lean proteins. After doing this for a while and the scale barely budged, I started calculating each gram of carbohydrates, proteins, and fats. Ultimately, I decided to implement a strict 40/40/20 ratio on a daily basis. This had worked in the past and it was the same program that helped my clients collectively lose thousands of pounds throughout the years. But, it was not working for me . . . and I created it.

After nearly a year, I was physically stronger and more emotionally balanced. However, when I looked in the mirror, the person I saw didn't reflect the strength I was gaining, the fitness level I was experiencing or the positive mindset I regained. In other words, my "healthy eating" choices weren't resulting in the body I hoped it would create. It seemed like the hours and months I spent exercising meant nothing. I was afraid all the years I spent trying to avoid my family history of diabetes and high blood pressure meant nothing as well. Consequently, I questioned whether or not I would end up suffering from these illnesses, too.

Something just didn't seem right. I was sure there was something wrong with me. So, I went to my doctor and asked her to run a complete metabolic panel, test my thyroid and anything else she believed would be beneficial. All test results came back normal for two years! My doctor simply said, "It just comes with age, you eat healthy, workout on a regular basis and you have no health issues so I'm not concerned." But, I was concerned because excess weight, even with a healthy lifestyle, eventually lead to illness*. I knew my healthy eating habits and active lifestyle were good methods to delay illness but my risk was still high.

When my tests all came back normal, this was the turning point for me. If there was nothing "wrong" with me, physically, there still had to be something happening within my body. So, I stopped blaming myself and started looking for solutions. I believed there had to be some other approach to weight loss.

I pulled out my old college textbooks and notes from my Exercise and Nutrition class. After flipping through chapter after chapter, I found a small section explaining ketogenic eating and how it changes the metabolic process of the body. It explained how it affected the body's ability to burn fat. FAT as fuel? I was intrigued. It was the opposite of everything I was taught to believe as the "best approach" for health and weight loss. Now, I discovered there was not just ONE way to lose weight and be healthy. I need to know more.

After spending the better part of a year delving into scientific research on ketogenic eating (which lead me to research intermittent fasting and eventually angiogenesis inhibiting foods), I had to unlearn many of the "truths" I thought I knew. For example, for years, I was told (and I repeated to others) fat was bad and wholegrain was the key to health. I also believed that breakfast was the "most important meal of the day" and I believed I had to eat every 3-4 hours to "boost my metabolism". But, in reality, all that advice was conditional and it didn't work for everyone.

After adopting ketogenic eating into my life, the first thing I noticed was my increased focus, energy, and productivity. Then, I stepped on the scale and the number started to decrease weekly. Soon, I lost 38lbs, reduced my body fat by15%, dropped 8 pant sizes and I kept it off! But even better than that, now, I wake up almost every morning feeling amazing. I am energized to start my day. I have mental clarity and focus. And, for the first time in a long time, I love the body I see when I look in the mirror because the person I see in the mirror is a reflection of the person I feel inside.

When I was writing my book, *The mR40 method: The 40 Day Guide to Reset Your Metabolism, Lose Weight and Optimize Your Health.* I chose to emphasize the ketogenic way of life, including information on how to do a complete Metabolic Reset in 40 Days. I also you to know you have the ability to change your physical and mental health for the better.

I understand there is no one diet for weight loss and my mR40 method may not be for everyone but if you...

- have been trying to lose weight and despite doing everything "right" the scale barely budges
- are feeling stuck in a cycle of trying, failing, trying and failing again
- exercise for hours just to feel exhausted and see no results
- struggle with food cravings, mood swings, and hormone imbalances and know it's related to your food but don't know where to start correcting it
- hate trying to lose weight means sticking to a diet that makes you 'hangy' and leaves you feeling defeated
- are tired of spending hours cooking and doing meal prep just to eat what amounts to microwaved "leftovers" because you are force feeding yourself every 3-4 hours.
- are sick and tired of feeling sick and tired

...then the mR40 method will teach you the science and research of how *to lose weight, balance your hormones, increase your energy, reduce inflammation and optimize your health in a practical and sustainable lifestyle.*

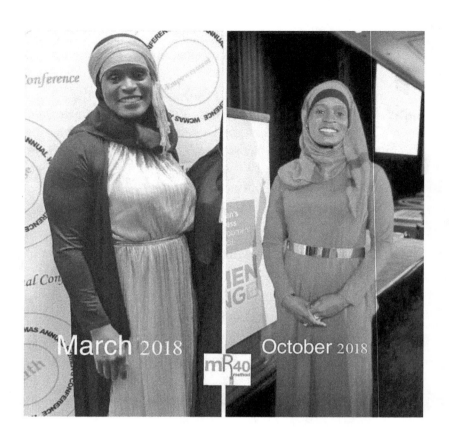

March 2018

October 2018

Welcome to Your 40-Day Metabolic Reset!

Over the next forty days, I am going to ask you to think differently about what certain foods, carbohydrates, fats, and proteins do for and to your body. For many, this book may be the line that connects the dots. For others, it may be a completely new way of thinking about your relationship with food. But as we begin to revamp your diet and lifestyle, based on the information in this book, you will not only lose weight and reshape your body; you will nourish your body in a way that will give you more energy, mental focus, and clarity, a stronger immune system and a resistance to disease.

I write this with understanding that for some people, this book is the last resort after years of yo-yo dieting, crash dieting, and exploring just to find yourself back at square one. For others, this is a kick-start to healthier eating, and for some others it's a way to get a better understanding of how your current healthy eating choices work on a physiological level.

On the other hand, you may be unsure why you picked up this book; all you know is that you feel sick, constipated, discouraged, depressed, overweight, and in need of a little guidance and encouragement so that you can fix whatever is weighing you down, physically and emotionally.

For each and every one of you, this can be a place to find what you need within these pages to help you restore your body, mind, and spirit.

Thank you for allowing me to join you on your journey of health and wellness.

Mubarakah Ibrahim

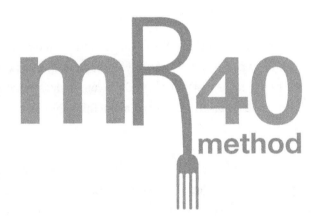

Chapter 1:

What is
the mR40 Method

When I developed the mR40 method, as a 40 day metabolic reset , I wanted to combine the most effective techniques for rapid weight loss in a way that makes them practical for anyone looking for a guaranteed method to shed excess fat while simultaneously improving their health. As a result of years of research and applying these methods to my own health and fitness journey and that of my clients, I created this program, which is based on four well-researched methods that have been scientifically proven to burn excess fat quickly and permanently while simultaneously improving various other health markers.

1. **Food Timing:** By consuming your calories in a specific, timed eating window, you will not only optimize how your body burns fat but also reduce inflammation, increase vitality, and detoxify your body on a cellular level.

2. **Macronutrient Manipulation:** Using a nutritional ketogenic-based eating plan, you will train your body to burn its own excess body fat as metabolic fuel. Once your body is adapted, I'll show you how to easily maintain this while enjoying delicious foods.

3. **Fat-Burning AI Foods:** Incorporating metabolic-enhancing, angiogenesis-inhibiting (AI) foods will encourage your body to reduce fat storage and maintain a healthy weight, allowing you to lose the weight AND keep it off.

4. **Metabolic Reconditioning Movement:** Strategically using high-intensity movements, you will burn more fat in a shorter amount of time, have a higher metabolism over a twenty-four-hour period, and improve your fitness level faster than any other form of exercise.

Each one of these techniques alone has been shown to be effective, but together they make an unstoppable formula to rapidly lose excess fat, increase energy, improve mental clarity, and boost overall health. The truth is, if you incorporated only one principle of this program into your everyday lifestyle, you would lose weight. If you added two principles to what you do on a daily basis, you would increase fat burn. When you incorporate all four aspects of the program together, the results are a program that creates a fat-burning inferno.

What Makes the mR40 Method Different from Other Keto Programs?

Ketogenic diets in general differ from Atkins by focusing on fat consumption and limiting protein. However, I've found that many ketogenic diets, even the fairly decent plans, are based solely on the macronutrient proportions with little concern given to the quality of the foods eaten. That's why you see so many keto meals using bacon and other processed meats. The mR40 method is not just about eating ketogenic; it's about getting the most benefit from the foods we eat and maximizing the advantages of being in a ketogenic state. Combining ketogenic eating with angiogenesis-inhibiting foods and metabolic-conditioning movements is the eugenics of weight loss plans.

What Makes the mR40 Method Different from Atkins?

Dr. Robert Atkins deserves credit for introducing low-carb eating to the mainstream. His method focused on limiting carbs—between twenty and twenty-five grams (g) of net carbs (total carbs minus fiber)—and eating protein, but provided little focus on fat consumption. The diet also didn't give much credence to the types of foods consumed, and as a result many people missed the mark on not just higher fat consumption but also the quality of the foods they ate, which is why Atkins is often characterized by loads of bacon and steak. Although it may sound great to eat all the bacon your heart desires, the problem, unfortunately, is that a low-carb, high-protein diet can actually prevent you from staying in nutritional ketosis because the body can convert protein into glucose through a process called gluconeogenesis, making it difficult to get into ketosis.

Why 40 Days and Not 21 Days?

Often, we hear it takes twenty-one days to create a habit. No one knows for sure exactly where this number came from. The best guess is a widely popular 1960 book called *Psycho-Cybernetics* by Maxwell Maltz, a plastic surgeon turned psychologist who noticed his patients seemed to take about twenty-one days to get used to their new faces.

In the preface to *Psycho-Cybernetics*, Dr. Maxwell Maltz wrote: "It usually requires a minimum of about twenty-one days to effect any perceptible change in a mental image. Following plastic surgery, it takes about twenty-one days for the average patient to get used to his new face. When an arm or leg is amputated the 'phantom limb' persists for about twenty-one days. People must live in a new house for about three weeks before it begins to seem like home. These and many other commonly observed phenomena tend to show that it requires a minimum of about twenty-one days for an old mental image to dissolve and a new one to jell" (pp. xiii-xiv).

But researchers have since studied different types of habit formation to figure out how long it actually takes to create a habit. In a study of ninety-six people over a twelve-week period at the University of London College,[1] each person chose one new habit for the twelve weeks and reported each day on whether they did the behavior and how automatic the behavior felt.

Researchers found that habit creation can vary from person to person based on the amount of effort it takes to complete the task. For example, participants whose habit was drinking water on a daily basis were able to create that habit much quicker than someone doing fifty sit-ups every day. Drinking water was a low barrier habit, where sit-ups required greater commitment,

---

[1] https://onlinelibrary.wiley.com/doi/abs/10.1002/ejsp.674

energy, and time. Researchers found that the length of time can vary from eighteen days for low barrier habits to as much as 264 days for more complex habits. However, the peak of habit building occurred around day forty.

In the past, I have recommended and even led clients through twenty-one-day diets and exercise programs. However, in my experience, most people do not make lasting change with just three weeks of behavior change. When the twenty-one days are over, they are very likely to go back to previous habits, giving more credence in my mind to the research that it takes longer than twenty-one days to make lasting change.

The type of lifestyle we live is composed of daily habits. From what we choose to eat— which is normally not a conscious effort but habitual patterns of food—to how we move and how we manage stress. During the mR40 method phase I, we are recreating your habits to restore your physical, mental, and emotional health. Committing to a forty-day plan not only allows you to break less healthy habits but also establish new ones that are much more likely to stick.

The History 40-Day Transformation

The designation of forty days has been a significant period of time that allows transformation, renewal, repair, regeneration, and rebirth to occur in both the physical and spiritual well-being for thousands of years across many faiths, cultures, and traditions.

According to Islamic history, the Prophet Muhammad (PBUH) would pray and fast in the cave of Hira for forty days to attain spiritual renewal before he received the divine message of prophethood. In Judaism, there's a mystical practice that says one who seeks an answer to their prayers should pray the same prayer request for forty consecutive days, and the Prophet Moses (PBUH) is believed to have spent forty days on Mount Sinai, where he received the Ten Commandments. Forty days also has significance for Christians who fast for forty days during Lent. In all the aforementioned Abrahamic faiths, it is also believed that when God sought to purify the world, the rains of the flood lasted for forty days and forty nights before the Prophet Noah and his people emerged from the Ark.

Within many other cultures and practices around the world, forty days also holds much significance in traditional practices. In China, Africa, and Latin America, a new mother is "confined" to her home for forty days after she has given birth, during which time she is cared for by family and visited by friends, and given time for her body to be restored, to bond with her baby, and to recuperate from her pregnancy and labor.

Even when we look at the physiology of the human body, we see renewal in many ways using a forty-day pattern. Adult skin cells, on average, take forty days to renew, and our red blood cells start dying from forty days onward to replace cells with new life-sustaining ones.

It's with this knowledge and tradition in mind that I developed the mR40 method: The 40-Day Metabolic Reset.

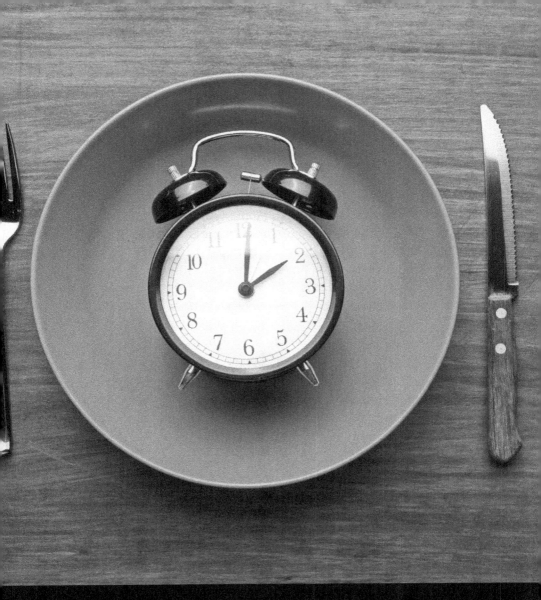

Chapter 2:

Eat, Stop, Eat:
Intermittent Fasting

Often when people ask me what is the one thing they can do to lose weight, my response is "Eat less." Not to be snarky (okay, maybe a little), but this is an honest answer. Most people in developed countries eat way too much, our portions are bigger than necessary for our sedentary lifestyle, and we also eat way too often.

A National Health and Nutrition Examination Survey (NHANES) states that 39.6 percent of American adults are obese, a significant rise in American obesity statistics from just ten years ago. The same NHANES data reports 41.1 percent of women and 37.9 of men are obese. But even more alarming is the prevalence of Class 3 obesity. Class 3 obesity is the CDC's term for people who are 100 pounds or more overweight, or with a BMI above 40. New research shows that about 8 percent of adults now fall into Class 3, up from less than 6 percent in 2007.

I believe in intermittent fasting as the first line of defense (and offense) against obesity and a wide range of health ills. Among the multitude of health benefits fasting provides, there are four main reasons I included intermittent fasting as a part of the mR40 method.

Number 1: It is the simplest way to jump-start fat burn. Simply skipping a meal can get your fat-burning gears turning and prime your body for weight loss.

Number 2: It both starts and accelerates ketosis and in essence hacks your keto diet to get faster results.

Number 3: It increases human growth hormone (HGH), which maintains and builds muscle. This paired with the mR40 exercise protocol can result in long-term increase of the metabolism by increasing muscle mass—allowing you to lose weight and keep it off permanently.

Number 4: It improves insulin sensitivity, leading to multitudes of health benefits, including reducing inflammation and staving off diabetes.

I wanted to include fasting as the first eating recommendation because it's the simplest to do, and it alone has been shown to increase weight loss and improve health.

A Historical View of Fasting

"Breakfast is the most important meal of the day." So we've been told and so we've repeated. Turns out that isn't the holy grail. If there is one habit I could encourage people to adopt to lose weight, it would be to stop eating "all the time." It sounds a bit tongue-in-cheek with an undertone of sarcasm, but honestly it's not. We have been convinced that eating three to five times a day is what we have to do to lose weight, and that's simply not true. In fact, historically human beings have not even had the ability to eat so often until the mechanical age of transportation and refrigeration.

As a practicing Muslim, once a year I spend thirty days going sixteen to eighteen hours a day not eating or drinking. (No, not even water.) The fast during the Islamic month of Ramadan dictates Muslims to stop eating and drinking during daylight hours and most Muslims feel physically healthier and more productive during this time.

Muslims are not the only group of people who fast by refraining from eating and/or drinking for extended periods of time. Chapter 2 verse 183 in the Holy Qur'an says (what is translated as), *"O ye who believe! Fasting is prescribed for you, even as it was prescribed for those before you, that ye may ward off (evil),"* recognizing spiritual revelations before the Quran was revealed to the Prophet Muhammad (PBUH) also instructed followers to fast as a sort of spiritual armament.

The Jewish calendar contains several fast days, including the twenty-five-hour fast of Yom Kippur—the Day of Atonement— which is considered the most important holiday in the Jewish faith. It marks the culmination of the Ten Days of Awe, a period of introspection and repentance that follows Rosh Hashanah, the Jewish New Year.

According to Christianity, fasts in Bible times were three days (Esther 4:16) or even seven days (1 Samuel 31:13). And on three occasions, fasts lasted forty days: Moses receiving the Ten Commandments (Exodus 34:28), Elijah encountering

God (1 Kings 19:8), and Jesus being tempted in the wilderness (Matthew 4).

However, fasting isn't limited to the Abrahamic faiths of Judaism, Christianity, and Islam. Many spiritual lifestyles and philosophies practice fasting, including Buddhism, Taoism, Jainism, and Hinduism. It has been used as a means of spiritual renewal, mental clarity, and physical cleansing for centuries. I believe part of this is due to the fact that fasting has physical benefits that enhance both how we feel physically and our clarity of thought. Those who fast report that the beneficial physical effects on their minds and bodies include mental clarity and a boost in energy levels, which have all been documented in research.

The physical effects are profound enough that fasting can be used as a means of improving overall health even if done for a short period of time or in periodic bursts. Researchers have been looking into the effects that various types of fasting have on the body, and the findings have been absolutely fascinating. Weight loss, increased mental focus and clarity, cellular detoxification, improved insulin sensitivity, and increased cellular regeneration are all effects of eating less often.

What Is Intermittent Fasting and How Is It Different from Starving?

Intermittent fasting is a deliberate eating method of going without food for a specific length of time during the day or week. It cycles between being in a fed state and a fasting state. It does not dictate which foods to eat but rather when you should eat. There are several different intermittent fasting methods, all of which split the day or week into eating periods and fasting periods. The following are several methods of intermittent fasting based on health goals and tolerance levels.

> 12:12 – Fasting for twelve hours a day and limiting eating time to a twelve-hour window. [Good start for beginners to introduce the body to the concept.]

16:8 – Fasting for sixteen hours a day and limiting eating time to an eight-hour window. [Most common way of fasting because of its practicality. Most often practiced by stopping eating at 8 p.m., skipping breakfast, and having the first meal at noon.]

20:4 – Fasting for twenty hours a day and limiting eating time to a four-hour window. [The most effective fast for weight loss since the greatest lipolysis happens between hours eighteen and twenty.]

5:2 – Fasting for twenty-four hours twice a week on non-consecutive days. [Effective for weight loss/maintenance and health with fewer daily restrictions.]

1:1 or Alternate Day Fasting – Fasting for twenty-four consecutive hours every other day.

36 hours – Going without food for thirty-six consecutive hours once a month, drinking only water, black coffee, and black/green tea. [Less common but effective for people who want a boost in brainpower and muscle growth.]

The important thing to remember is that intermittent fasting is a diet, not an eating pattern. It's not intended as a method of starvation or even calorie reduction, although that can be a side effect. But even when you eat the equivalent calories and macronutrients, fasting produces more weight loss than simple calorie reduction on a non-fasting diet.

How Does Intermittent Fasting Help with Weight Loss?

Using intermittent fasting alone is an effective weight loss strategy, even without ketogenic eating or other calorie-cutting, higher carb plans. In several studies done by UK researcher Michelle Harvie, comparing intermittent fasting to traditional calorie-cutting diets, fasting has been repeatedly shown to outperform traditional diets in terms of weight loss, reduction in body fat, and improved insulin resistance.

We used to believe that going more than three or four hours without food would slow down the metabolism. Now we know that's simply not true. When done properly, short-term dietary fasting is the absolute 100 percent quickest (and healthiest) way possible to strip your body of stubborn body fat.

Some people might argue that skipping meals goes against our better judgment. Others are unsure about getting all the nutrients, vitamins, and minerals they need during a fast, but to all of those people, I say ask yourself: *Did our ancestors have food readily available at all times? Did cavemen have refrigerators?* Of course not! Our bodies are highly intelligent biological machines even without our conscious effort. Periodic fasting has been a natural cycle of our existence since the beginning of human existence.

Stop Starving: Ghrelin and Leptin

Once you are adapted to this method of eating, you don't have to count calories because not many people overeat with intermittent fasting (you are just not that hungry), and that's why this eating pattern is so great. It helps us stick to the diet we are already on.

The hardest part of any "diet plan" is feeling like you are *on a diet.* This is the main cause for most people not sticking to their dietary choices. "I feel like I'm always starving" is a common complaint I hear. But it's not your fault and it's not from a lack of willpower and no, you are not "just greedy." Because low-calorie, carb-based diet plans fluctuate your insulin levels, they also trigger a fluctuation in your "hunger hormones," making you feel hungry, sometimes even when you are not.

Ghrelin and leptin are known as our "eating hormones." Ghrelin is called the "hunger hormone" because it stimulates appetite and promotes fat storage. It is produced and released primarily by the stomach (although very small amounts are also released by the small intestine, pancreas, and brain). When your stomach is empty, your body produces ghrelin, which travels to the hypothalamus in the brain to signal you are hungry, and tells your body to stop burning calories and store energy as fat.

Leptin, on the other hand, is referred to as the "satiety hormone." It decreases appetite by signaling the brain's hypothalamus to tell your body to stop eating and your metabolism to kick it up a notch. Leptin is secreted primarily in fat cells, as well as the stomach, heart, placenta, and skeletal muscles. Its main role is to prevent us from overeating and regulate how much fat we carry on our bodies. It also has many other functions related to immunity, brain function, and fertility. The more fat cells you have, the higher the leptin levels and the more satisfied you feel between meals.

Unfortunately, that doesn't always result in decreased appetite, particularly for people who are obese. Like insulin resistance, where the body stops responding to insulin signaling over time, our body can also become leptin resistant and stop responding to the overproduction of leptin caused by excess fat cells. Both ghrelin and leptin are very responsive to not just eating but the insulin response after we eat.

Fasting improves insulin sensitivity and maintains insulin stability, reducing fluctuation that may create false hormonal signals. This makes it easier to fast without feeling like you are starving.

If you are hesitant to begin and want to start slowly incorporating intermittent fasting, I recommend starting with a twelve-hour fast. Give your body twelve hours between dinner and breakfast every single day for a week. The liver depletes its glycogen stores after a twelve-hour fast and will begin burning fat as fuel. After following this twelve-hour eating pattern for a week, extend the fast anywhere from sixteen to twenty hours a day depending on your goals and tolerance level.

An average sixteen-hour fasting day would mean that you stop eating at 8 p.m. and eat your first meal at noon the next day. Simply put, it's skipping breakfast and making lunch your first meal. Drinking black coffee, unsweetened green or black tea, and water during the morning is fine. The general rule is not to consume any more than about fifty calories to prevent your body's digestive metabolism from fully kicking in and reducing the health and fat-burning advantage of the fast. Once your digestive tract activates, this begins a series of chemical and hormonal responses that change your body into a fed state and breaks your fast.

For people who work at night and sleep during the day, the fast can also be reversed as long as it's done in consecutive hours. For example, if you sleep during the day from 9 a.m. to 4 p.m., then you would have your last meal at 7 a.m., leaving two hours for digestion before bed, and eat your first meal at 7 p.m. on a twelve-hour fast.

Fat Loss by Any Other Name: Lipolysis

As the glycogen is depleted from the liver after twelve hours of going without food, insulin levels also drop significantly. This drop in insulin opens the door for a reduction in fat storage and an increase in fat burn, in part due to the increase in human growth hormone (HGH), which is the mother of all fat-burning hormones. But the twelve-hour mark is just the tip of the iceberg. According to research by Ted Naiman, M.D., "the sweet spot" for intermittent fasting occurs between eighteen and twenty-four hours of fasting, since this is the time period that sees the greatest drop in insulin and increase in lipolysis, the technical term for our body-burning fat, which means that our bodies are the most efficient at burning fat for fuel after almost a day of not eating.

Furthermore, when insulin decreases, it signals the body to increase the production of HGH. It appears the lower the insulin dips, the higher production of HGH, which is why longer fasts result in greater amounts of HGH. Researchers at the Intermountain Medical Center Heart Institute found that men who had fasted for twenty-four hours had a 2,000 percent increase in circulating HGH. Women who were tested had a 1,300 percent increase in HGH. It's important to note that this doesn't mean going without food for weeks raises HGH much higher. After thirty-six hours most hormonal responses level off.

But the benefits of HGH don't stop there...

Muscle Is As Muscle Does

One of the biggest challenges for weight loss programs is to allow the body to maximize burning stored fat while minimizing the loss of precious muscle fibers. This has always been a challenge even for the most informed trainer and coach. The metabolism is directly related to how much muscle you have. For every pound of muscle you gain, you increase your metabolism by about fifty calories a day. The reverse is also true—for every pound of muscle you lose, you decrease your metabolism by about fifty calories a day. Many weight loss programs allow the scale to decrease, but because part of that decrease is muscle, it's harder to maintain the weight loss as the metabolism becomes slower, creating a double-edged sword. You have a slower metabolism, so you have to eat less, and eating less creates the psychological stress of never being able to enjoy high-calorie foods without it resulting in weight gain. This is what I call the "donut effect": when clients feel like if they even smell a donut, they gain weight.

An increase in HGH has been shown not only to increase the body's ability to burn fat but also maintain and build muscle at the same time, making it easier to lose the weight when fasting *and* keep it off. This fact is what debunks the myth that intermittent fasting causes you to lose muscle.

As an added perk, there is strong evidence that HGH stimulates collagen synthesis (i.e., increases the glue that binds and strengthens our muscles) and improves the function and strength of muscles, tendons, ligaments, bones, and exercise performance as a result. In other words, get ready to **SMASH YOUR FITNESS GOALS.** These increases will allow you to go faster and lift heavier while minimizing risk of injury.

But wait—there's more…

Anti-Inflammatory: Human Growth Hormone

As I pointed out, human growth hormone (HGH) and insulin functions oppose one another: HGH is focused on tissue repair, efficient fuel usage, and anti-inflammatory immune activity. Insulin is designed for energy storage, cellular division, and pro-inflammatory immune activity. Fasting increases HGH and decreases insulin, consequently reducing the inflammatory state of the body, which improves brain function and overall tissue healing. This is extremely important because inflammation is one of the leading underlying causes of disease.

As scientists delve deeper into the fundamental causes of illnesses like type 2 diabetes, coronary artery disease, Alzheimer's, and even certain cancers like colon cancer, they are starting to see links to the immunological defense mechanism called inflammation—the same biological process that turns the tissue around a paper cut red and causes swelling in an injured toe. The reduction of inflammation may be one of the primary ways to improve your health and increase vitality and longevity.

All adults have some level of chronic inflammation slowly waging a war on our tissues and organs, and its activity is only detected in blood tests. But if it's turned up a notch or two, chronic inflammation can wear away at the body, causing devastating damage.

What Is Inflammation?

There are two main types of inflammation: acute inflammation and chronic inflammation. We experience inflammation on a regular basis, so many people are familiar with it as a concept.

Acute inflammation happens when we stomp our toe or get bitten by a mosquito and our body creates a barrier of "inflammation"—primarily by sending white blood cells to localize the problem. It brings the body's immune cells, hormones, and nutrients to the area to fix the problem. It's like an army that surrounds an invading enemy not just to neutralize them but also contain them so that they do not affect the rest of the population.

We see the result of "army activity" by redness, swelling, and pain. White blood cells flow into the injured area and destroy germs, dead or damaged cells, and other foreign materials, and help heal the body.

Like many other functions in our body, the inflammation process is a protective mechanism that goes awry when it happens too often or for a prolonged period of time. *Too much of a good thing is not a good thing.* When the inflammation process is triggered on a consistent basis from things like the toxins we come in contact with, the foods we eat, or the excess hormones produced from toxic stress, it causes a chain reaction and results in *chronic inflammation.*

Chronic inflammation, sometimes called persistent or low-grade inflammation, on the other hand, happens when the body gets a "false alarm" and sends the same inflammatory response to a perceived internal threat that does not require an inflammatory response. The white blood cells swarm the area, but have nothing to do and nowhere to go, and they eventually start attacking other tissues and cells, resulting in conditions as debilitating as arthritis or as serious as lupus. These are called autoimmune diseases and are the result of chronic inflammation.

It's like a fire truck being called to a house and told there is a fire in the walls. There is no fire but the firemen (white blood cells) begin to knock down doors, ax open the Sheetrock, and remove beams in search of a fire that doesn't exist. The biggest problem is that chronic inflammation can go on forever, slowly and silently chipping away at our health.

Chronic inflammation is not just the cause of more serious autoimmune diseases like lupus; it also plays a primary role in a host of other illnesses—in part due to the body producing what researchers at Yale School of Medicine refer to as inflammasome, specifically NLRP3, which drives the inflammatory response in several disorders, including type 2 diabetes, Alzheimer's disease, atherosclerosis, and even cancer.

Healthy lifestyle habits such as exercising regularly, not smoking, maintaining a healthy weight, and minimizing stress all help to reduce inflammation. But one of the biggest factors in chronic, low-level inflammation may be the food you eat every day. When we consider the ways to create the biggest impact on our health, preventing inflammation is a pathway to better health as well as a better quality of life.

The good news is that endogenous metabolites, also known as "ketone bodies"—a compound produced by the body called β-hydroxybutyrate (BHB)—inhibit these inflammasomes. In a research study published in the online issue of *Nature Medicine*,[2] a team of Yale University scientists, working with mice and human immune cells, introduced BHB to mouse models of inflammatory diseases. They found that this introduction of ketone bodies markedly reduced inflammation. Inflammation was also reduced when the mice were given a ketogenic diet, which elevates the levels of BHB in the bloodstream.

BHB is naturally produced by the body in response to three things: fasting, a low-carb, ketogenic diet, or high-intensity exercise, all of which are a part of the mR40 method.

Intermittent Fasting Terms

Before we go further, let's define some of the main terms for the purpose of the mR40 method program.

Fasting: Going more than twelve hours without the consumption of any food or drink that collectively has a caloric value above fifty or causes a significant digestive or hormonal response. [For example, adding one tablespoon. of heavy cream to coffee (45 calories / 0 glycemic response) does not break the fast, but adding three-quarters of a tablespoon of honey that has a high insulin response will break the fast (45 calories / 100 glycemic response).]

---

[2] https://www.nature.com/articles/nm.3804

Wet Fasting: Going more than twelve hours without the consumption of any foods. Water, black coffee, and tea are allowed.

Dry Fasting: Going more than twelve hours without the consumption of any food or caloric beverages. NO water, coffee, or black tea is allowed. [Muslim fast of Ramadan and Jewish fast of Yom Kippur]

Intermittent Fasting [IF]: A schedule of eating where you are engaging in wet fasting or dry fasting for a predetermined amount of time, allowing yourself a certain window of time during which you consume all calories for the day.

Fed Window: Refers to the hours in the day that you are eating and digesting food.

Fasting Window: Refers to the consecutive hours of the day you are not eating.

mR40 Intermittent Fasting

Starting your journey with a complete twenty-four-hour "wet fast" is recommended to get you in both a physical and mental state in which to embark on your new lifestyle journey. This one-day initial fast will prime your body and your mind to the concept of change. It may be uncomfortable and even hard for some people, but challenging yourself and moving outside of your comfort zone is a part of the journey of becoming a better you.

Jump-start

During your twenty-four hours, stay hydrated by drinking plenty of water. If you have an energy slump, consume black coffee or green tea with no sugar or cream. Counter to what you may think, make sure you have plans or work during the day. Staying busy will prevent you from thinking about food and feeling hungry.

Phase I

Day 2 you will enter Phase I of the mr40 method program where you fast sixteen to twenty hours every day depending on your goals and tolerance level. This may seem like a long time if you have not done extended fasts before; however, intermittent fasting paired with ketogenic eating makes going extended periods of time not only easy but more beneficial for both methods. Fat and protein produce a feeling of satiety, so the combination of high fat and moderate protein levels with ketogenic eating suppresses the appetite. This is the result of three key hormone changes. Fasting causes insulin levels to drop, and like a domino effect, this creates a reaction of ghrelin and leptin levels, which regulate your hunger as explained earlier in this chapter.

The added benefit that many people who adopt intermittent fasting realize is how free they feel. Simply not being confined to a three- to four-hour eating schedule gives one a level of being unchained for being a slave to food. And because meals are not as frequent, spending hours meal-prepping becomes completely unnecessary.

Phase II

This phase is after you have completed the first forty days OR when you have reached your goal weight and fasting is used to improve and maintain overall health more than weight management. In phase II you will fast for twenty to twenty-four hours twice a week on non-consecutive days. Ketone bodies produced by fasting promote positive changes in the structure of synapses important for learning and overall brain health. In addition, research is showing it might help your brain ward off neurodegenerative diseases like Alzheimer's and Parkinson's while at the same time improving memory and mood.

During the fast you can consume:

Water (minimum of half your body weight in ounces of water daily)

Black coffee (NO creams, sweeteners, or sugar substitutes)

Black / green tea (NO creams, sweeteners, or sugar substitutes)

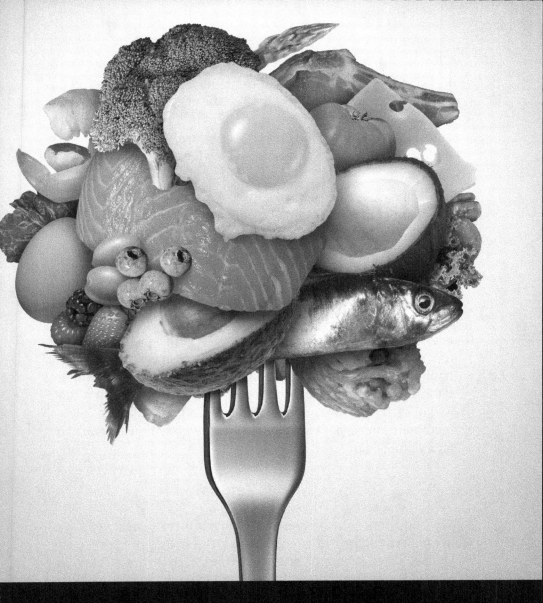

Chapter 3:

Key To What?
Ketosis Explained

Using food and food timing to get your metabolic system to switch to ketosis is the second eating method in this program. But before we get into how to use food as a method of being in ketosis, I want you to fully understand the physiological process of how ketosis was discovered and how it actually works.

Ketosis is like a fasting hack. Seriously, that's not just a catchphrase. It was actually discovered as a way to get the benefits of fasting without actually fasting. Fasting was used to reduce seizures in pediatric patients, but preventing patients from eating was not a practical (or healthy) long-term strategy. In the process of trying to figure out the physiological changes that happen with fasting, altering the brain enough to stop seizures, scientists discovered that during fasting, the body metabolizes fat stores and then the fatty acids undergo beta-oxidation into acetoacetate, β-hydroxybutyrate, and acetone—ketone bodies the cell can then use as precursors to generate adenosine triphosphate (ATP)—our body's energy source. Scientists then figured out the same process can be induced by eating a diet low in carbohydrates and very high in fats to simulate the same metabolic effects of fasting by forcing the body to use primarily fat as a fuel source.

What Is Ketosis?

The body prefers to use glucose because it is the easiest molecule to convert and use as energy. In fact, the body's preference for glucose takes such a priority that when carbohydrate intake is low and protein intake is high, it will even manage to convert the amino acids in protein into glucose, a process called gluconeogenesis. This is the reason people who follow low-carb/high-protein diets have a difficult time getting into ketosis and seeing the weight loss results they were hoping for. Too much protein in the diet will produce enough glucose to prevent ketosis. Because anytime the body is able to create energy from glucose, it will NOT convert fat into ketones for energy.

This is a common misconception about keto diets, and it produces terms like "keto light" and "modified keto diet" when in actuality there is no such thing. One can reduce one's carbohydrates and avoid added sugars for a healthier diet; however, it is not a keto diet because the body is not using ketones for energy. To truly be a ketogenic diet, the body's response must be a physiological state of ketosis. This can physically be measured through urine, blood, or breath analyzers as we will discuss later.

How Does a Ketogenic Diet Actually Work?

The best way to understand how ketosis actually works is to imagine the body like a house that needs an electrical supply of energy. Remember, energy is not only what you need to run, jump, and lift weights; every function of your body requires energy for you to stay alive, to keep your heart beating, your lungs breathing, and your digestive system functioning.

For our analogy consider that most houses receive energy from electrical power grids that send electricity across power lines and into the house. Think of the electrical grids as a food source of carbohydrates. And carbohydrates aren't just grains like rice and bread or sweets like cookies and cakes; in fact most foods, with the exception of animal proteins and pure fats, contain some carbohydrates, including fruits, vegetables, legumes, and nuts. Our body converts all those carbohydrates into glucose for energy. Glucose for our analogy is the electrical current the grid sends across the power lines to produce energy for the house.

As an alternative all houses (bodies) have a backup generator that turns on when there are little to no electrical currents (carbohydrates) coming in. Think of the generator as ketosis and instead of electricity (glucose), it uses diesel fuel to produce energy for the house. The diesel fuel needed is fat. The generator gets its fuel (fat) from both our excess body fat and the fat we consume on a keto diet.

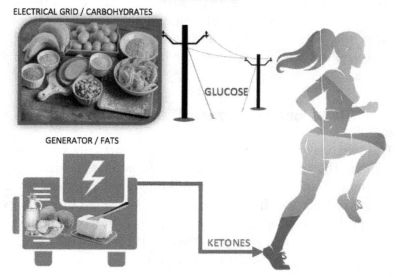

THIS IS HOW KETOSIS WORKS
mR40method.com

When electrical lines are cut (reducing carbohydrates), the generator (ketosis) kicks in automatically to produce energy. The body cannot simultaneously use both glucose and ketones as a main energy source, just as a house will not use electrical lines AND the generator simultaneously.

How Does Ketosis Help You Lose Weight?

When your body no longer relies on glucose, it looks for fat to convert to ketones to use as energy. The most abundant and accessible form of fat is your own stored body fat. When the process of ketosis is activated, the body releases its fat cells, which are converted into ketones for energy. But that's just part of the process of what makes being in a ketogenic state so beneficial for weight loss.

By significantly reducing carbohydrates you also reduce insulin, which is a fat storage hormone. When insulin drops it signals your body to stop storing fat. Simultaneously human growth hormone is released, which then signals your body to release stored fat. All these things together create the best possible scenario to burn excess fat storage.

The Domino Effect: Insulin

I refer to insulin as the "domino" hormone. When insulin is out of whack, it creates a domino effect that results in many of the diseases we mentioned earlier. That same insulin hormone is a big lighthouse signal attracting health pirates.

One of the main effects of excess insulin is fat storage. When insulin levels rise it signals the body to store fat instead of burn it, leading to excess body fat and obesity.

I believe the most important health benefit that fasting and ketogenic eating provide for many people is the effect on insulin sensitivity or how the body both produces and responds to insulin. When the body goes more than twelve hours without food, the first thing that happens is insulin levels drop. Insulin is a hormone produced in your pancreas when your body signals that you have eaten.

Here is how it works: When you eat, your body breaks down your food into glucose (the body's sugar), which flows into your bloodstream to transport nutrients into your cells for use as energy. This is significant because insulin is a pivotal hormone that can begin many other hormonal and metabolic responses, which is why I call insulin the domino hormone.

What is Insulin?

Insulin is a hormone that is secreted by the pancreas into the bloodstream to help transport nutrients and glucose throughout your body for use. After a meal, the digestive tract breaks down carbohydrates and converts them into glucose. Glucose is then absorbed into your bloodstream through the lining in your small intestine. Once glucose is in your bloodstream, insulin's main job is to allow the nutrients you eat into the cells to create energy.

Insulin is not bad. It's natural and necessary for our body. It's required for nutrients to get to the cells, for muscles to grow, but like with all other things, too much of a good thing is never a good thing.

How Does Insulin Work?

To understand how insulin works, let's use the analogy of a parking attendant at an airport parking garage. Each time a car (glucose) arrives, the parking attendant (insulin) opens the parking gate, allows the car (glucose) into the garage (cells), and directs it to the proper parking lot, either short-term (muscles) or mid-term parking (liver) or long term (fat cells). Our muscles can store approximately 500g of glucose in the form of glycogen and the liver can only store about 100g. When we have more glucose than our muscles and liver can store, the excess is converted into fat by the liver and stored as fat cells—i.e., sending cars to long-term parking—and there is no limit to the number of fat cells the human body can hold. In essence long-term parking is an a black whole with limitless space.

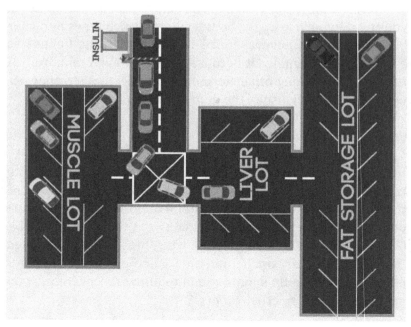

The mR40 Method

Insulin's job is to help balance your blood glucose levels or prevent a traffic backup of cars waiting to park. Insulin resistance is when the parking attendant can't open the gate to allow cars in because it's stuck from overuse. Insulin basically tries to unlock the cell to deliver the glucose, but the cell door won't open. As a result the pancreas sends more and more insulin to try to get the cell doors open, and this causes higher insulin levels, higher blood sugar levels, and leads to type 2 diabetes. In other words diabetes is when the parking gate is stuck and can't let cars in.

The problem with insulin is that it is a "fat storage" hormone and creates a domino effect of weight gain, inflammation, and a whole host of other unhealthful effects. (More on that in the chapter about insulin and weight gain.)

When you significantly reduce your dietary carbohydrates, your body cannot produce enough glucose for energy and it shifts into an "auxiliary" energy mode to where the body produces ketones from the breakdown of fats in the liver to be used as energy. This is called ketosis.

Health Effects of Ketosis That Will Change Your Life

Although you are probably looking for a weight loss plan, the mR40 method, which prioritizes being in ketosis, is so much more. The ways that ketosis benefit your health will not just help you look better but make you feel better physically, mentally, and even spiritually.

Cellular Detox: Autophagy

The dictionary definition of detox is to "abstain from or rid the body of toxic or unhealthy substances." The original layman's detox was related to ridding the body of drugs or alcohol in a medically supervised environment. But the word "detox" has crossed from medical intervention to prevention and wellness. The word has gained popularity over the last few years in the alternative health and wellness circles. Every "guru" has a different version of what they define as a detox—a word that's been used to describe everything from water fasting to juicing to eating meats and greens for thirty days.

The idea that we can CAUSE our body to detox is a myth. We are not some big ball of toxins that's simply waiting to implode into sickness and disease as many would lead you to believe. In fact our body is designed so we do not become overloaded with toxins. The truth is our body is always detoxing. We have seven ways in which our body detoxifies on a continual basis.

1. **The lungs** help the body releases gaseous wastes such as carbon dioxide. Proper breathing plays an important role in detoxification because it helps the body return to a relaxed state, when the body's detoxification systems are most active. Practicing deep breathing techniques is beneficial during the detoxification process.

2. **The lymphatic system** (composed of lymph nodes and the vessels that connect them) are another filtration system in the body for waste products. Enhancing the flow of lymph supports the body's ability to detoxify. Massage and dry skin brushing will help increase lymphatic flow.

3. **The kidney** is responsible for filtering blood and removing waste products from your body through urination. Kidneys are bean-shaped organs, each about the size of a fist located just below the rib cage, one on each side of your spine. The kidney's efficiency is partly affected by your hydration status and blood pressure. If either of these isn't optimal, toxins are more likely to circulate through your body instead of being eliminated.

4. **The colon** removes toxins and waste products through bowel movements. If you're not pooping regularly, toxins can remain in the colon for prolonged periods of time and can be reabsorbed back into your body.

5. **The skin** is the largest organ in the body. It provides a route for toxins to exit the body mainly through sweat and oil glands. Exercise and saunas are great ways to get the body sweating, encouraging the release of toxic buildup.

6. **The liver** is unlike the other organs mentioned above, in that it doesn't directly remove toxins from the body. However,

it plays a major role in detoxification pathways. It alters the chemistry of toxins it encounters so that they are more easily removed from the body. Eating foods higher in sulfur—such as beets, garlic, leafy greens, and green tea—supports the liver.

7. **Autophagy,** or cellular detoxification, is a metabolic process of genetic recycle and repair. It is literally detoxification on a cellular level through a process very similar to our *reduce, recycle, and reuse* mantra. It reduces unwanted and damaged cells and recycles broken cells so they can be reused to repair and regenerate newer cells.

The word "autophagy" goes back to 1974 when it was first used by Christian de Duve, but the scientific importance and understanding of it was highlighted when the 2016 Nobel Prize in Physiology or Medicine was awarded to Yoshinori Ohsumi for his discoveries of mechanisms for autophagy. There is a lot about the process and all the ways it affects the body that is still not completely understood because it's a relatively new area of research, but we do know a few very important health benefits of autophagy.

Even if you live a reasonably healthy lifestyle, the cells in your body are continually becoming damaged as a natural part of several metabolic processes. And as you get older and are exposed to more free radical damage, your cells become damaged at an increased rate. Over time, damaged cells can accumulate in the body and increase your risk of autoimmune diseases, infections, cardiomyopathy, liver disease, diabetes, cancer, neurodegeneration, and other unwanted conditions like inflammation.

The cleansing of autophagy is catabolic in nature; in fact autophagy is the Greek word for "self-eating," because it tears down old damaged cells to make room for new ones. By cleaning out the damaged cells and proteins in your body, autophagy helps you naturally detox, reduce inflammation, and maintain optimal health. Getting rid of these risks before they cause problems is essential to your physical well-being.

How does autophagy work?

Brain Boost. Mental Focus and Clarity

Although I rarely talk to clients who want to lose weight to improve mental clarity, it's always a side note. Mental focus and enhanced brain function as a result of fasting are due to the increase in brain-derived neurotrophic factor (BDNF), which has been called a "master molecule" and referred to as "Miracle-Gro for the brain" by Harvard neuropsychiatrist John J. Ratey, MD, author of *Spark, The Revolutionary New Science of Exercise and the Brain* (a book I LOVE and highly recommend).

Mental focus

Ketones are a neuroprotective antioxidant, which means they are like the brain's personal bodyguards. They have been found to act as an antioxidant, preventing harmful reactive oxygen species from damaging brain cells.

Ketones trigger the expression of brain-derived neurotrophic factor (BDNF), a protein that acts on specific neurons throughout the nervous system and the development of synapses and various lines of communication within the brain. Think of it like a superhighway: BDNF creates more exits and lanes, allowing faster and more efficient travel of information. Higher levels of BDNF lead to healthier neurons and better communication processes between neuroglial cells, contributing to better learning, memory, and mental focus. The benefit starts at twelve hours; however, some research has shown that fasting up to thirty-six hours has been shown to boost BDNF levels by up to 400 percent. Higher levels of BDNF lead to healthier neurons and better communication processes between these neuroglial cells, contributing to better learning, memory, and mental focus.

Type 1 diabetics who experience reduced cognitive function because of low blood sugar see those deficits erased by increasing β-hydroxybutyrate (BHB) through dietary medium chain triglycerides (the same fats found in coconut oil). In memory-impaired adults, some with Alzheimer's, BHB improved cognition. Scores improved in (rough) parallel with rising ketones. MCT oil (exogenous ketones) improved cognition in patients with mild to moderate Alzheimer's. A very low-carb diet improved memory in older adults. Again, ketones tracked with improvements.

Fountain of Youth?

Free radicals are chemically reactive molecules which can bind to our cells and cause damage and inflammation to cellular DNA and other proteins.

A ketogenic diet reduces oxidative damage within the body and increases the production of uric acid and other potent antioxidants.

Ketosis supports mitochondrial function by increasing mitochondrial glutathione, an important antioxidant that works directly within the mitochondria. This is important because orally ingested antioxidants such as those in our food don't make it into the mitochondria very easily.

I encourage you to further explore the research that continues to show that eating a ketogenic diet and restricting carbs can help a wide range of conditions, including:

- Epilepsy
- Type 2 Diabetes
- Type 1 Diabetes
- High Blood Pressure
- Alzheimer's Disease
- Parkinson's Disease
- Chronic Inflammation
- Autism

- Depression
- Heart Disease
- Polycystic Ovary Syndrome (POS)
- Fatty Liver Disease
- Cancer
- Migraines

Keto Terms

Ketones is a type of acid produced in the liver, made from fat that the body can use for energy. We all have ketones, whether we have diabetes or not. Ketones are chemicals made in the liver. In the absence of glucose, your body send ketones to your bloodstream so your muscles and other tissues can then use them for fuel. Ketones, also known as "ketone bodies," are byproducts of the body breaking down fat for energy that occurs when carbohydrate intake is low.

Ketosis is a natural process the body initiates to help us survive when food intake is low. During this state, we produce ketones, which are produced from the breakdown of fats in the liver. A ketogenic diet reduces carbohydrates, NOT calories, to shift the body into the state of ketosis. Ketosis is scientifically determined by the metabolic state of having ketones in the blood, typically above 0.5mmol/L. The purpose of a ketogenic diet is to eat in such a way (high fat, moderate protein, low carb) that it induces your body into ketosis.

Ketogenic refers to the physical state of metabolizing ketones for energy.

Ketoacidosis – Excessive ketone bodies can produce a dangerously toxic level of acid in the blood, called ketoacidosis. During ketoacidosis, the kidneys begin to excrete ketone bodies along with body water in the urine, causing some fluid-related weight loss. Ketoacidosis most often occurs in individuals with type 1 diabetes because they do not produce insulin, a hormone that prevents the overproduction of ketones. However, in a few rare cases, ketoacidosis has been reported to occur in nondiabetic individuals following a prolonged, very low-carbohydrate diet.

Ketogenic diet is a high-fat, low-carb, moderate-protein dietary approach.

Medical ketogenic diet: Very low-carb (under 5 percent) and high-fat (over 75 percent) diet used to treat medically diagnosed illnesses such as drug-resistant epilepsy and cancer.

Dietary or nutritional ketogenic diet is a ketogenic diet used for weight loss and/or health benefit. The macronutrient content of the nutritional ketogenic diet has between 5 to 15 percent carbohydrates and 60 to 75 percent fat content and protein under 20 percent.

Keto diet is a term used to describe eating with the goal of putting the body in a ketogenic state most if not all of the time.

Fat adapted is a term used when a person has been following a ketogenic diet for several months and their metabolism has adjusted to ketones as the default fuel for energy.

Metabolic Flexibility: The   ability to switch between carbohydrate metabolism and fat metabolism with relative ease. A person with metabolic flexibility can burn carbs when they eat them instead of storing them as fat and burn fat as fuels when carbohydrates are not available. Once you achieve metabolic flexibility you will be able to go in and out of ketosis after "flexing" in less time with little to no adverse effects.

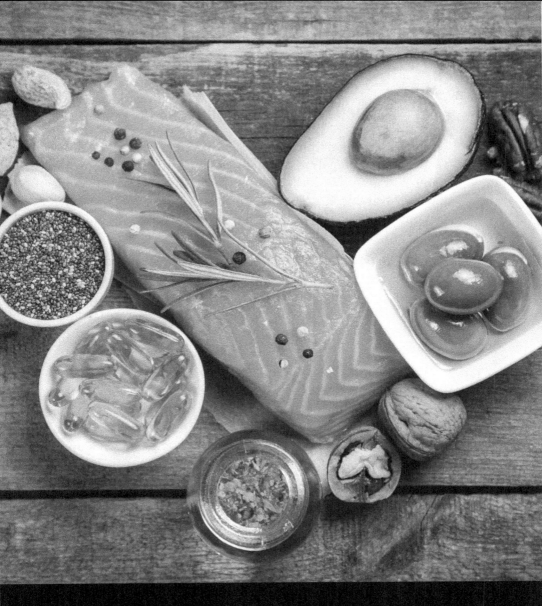

Chapter 4:

Got Fat?

What Is Ketogenic Eating and Why Do You Want to Do It?

The average American diet contains between 50 percent and 75 percent carbohydrates. That means on average men consume about 296 grams of carbohydrates a day and women consume about 224 grams of carbohydrates a day. These carbohydrates are converted into glucose, which the body metabolizes and uses as energy.

The ketogenic diet method changes the proportion of macronutrients to consuming most of your calories from fat (60 to 80 percent), a moderate amount of protein (15 to 20 percent), and a low amount of carbohydrates (below 15 percent), and as a result your body switches from burning glucose as fuel for energy to using fat.

When you significantly reduce your dietary carbohydrates, you will no longer produce enough glucose for your body to rely on for energy. In absence of glucose your body shifts to what I refer to as your "auxiliary" metabolism. The liver breaks down both dietary fat and stored fat into ketone bodies. When ketone bodies accumulate in the blood, this is called ketosis. Healthy individuals naturally experience a mild ketosis during periods of fasting (e.g., sleeping overnight) and after vigorous exercise.

The brain demands the most glucose in a steady supply, about 120 grams daily, because it cannot store glucose, unlike the liver and muscles. When very few carbohydrates are eaten, the body first pulls stored glucose from the liver and temporarily breaks down muscle to release glucose. If this continues for three or four days and stored glucose is fully depleted, blood levels of a hormone called insulin decrease, and the body begins to use fat as its primary fuel.

What is Ketoacidosis?

Much controversy has surrounded ketoacidosis and a ketogenic diet. Many people do not understand the science or physiology of how the process of metabolic reconditioning works when switching from glucose to ketones as a metabolic fuel source—and this can scare people away from adapting a ketogenic lifestyle. Ketoacidosis shouldn't be confused with being in the state of ketosis, which is harmless.

Ketoacidosis, however, is a harmful and life-threatening state that can occur when blood sugar levels are very high and insulin levels are low. As a result too many ketones build up, and the blood becomes acidic. Type 1 diabetics are at the highest risk of developing what is known as diabetic ketoacidosis (DKA) and are not encouraged to attempt a ketogenic diet unless specifically recommended and closely monitored by a medical professional.

Symptoms of diabetic ketoacidosis can appear quickly and may include one or more of the following symptoms:

- frequent urination
- extreme thirst
- high blood sugar levels
- high levels of ketones in the urine
- nausea or vomiting
- abdominal pain
- confusion
- fruity-smelling breath
- a flushed face
- fatigue
- rapid breathing
- dry mouth and skin

If you have type 1 diabetes and have a blood sugar reading of over 250 milligrams per deciliter (mg/dL), you should test your urine for ketones. Call your doctor if moderate or high levels of ketones are present. DKA is a medical emergency that can lead to a coma or death if left untreated. Call your local emergency services immediately if you think you are experiencing ketoacidosis.

Should I be Concerned About Ketoacidosis?

If you are NOT a type 1 diabetic, then following a well-formulated ketogenic eating plan will typically produce enough insulin to prevent excessive ketones from forming and blood levels of ketones reaching harmful level, and DKA and is not a major concern. Even those with type 2 diabetes are at very low risk for DKA because the body will produce enough insulin to prevent harmful drops in insulin levels and simultaneously improve insulin sensitivity, thus improving overall diabetic conditions.

Where Did the Ketogenic Diet Come From?

Because of the recent diet craze around ketogenic eating, many people think it's a new fad, but ketogenic eating is probably as old as human beings themselves. And the research around ketogenic eating dates back to the early twentieth century.

The historical theory: During Paleolithic times, which lasted from 2.6 million years ago to about 12,000 years ago, human beings hunted and gathered food. If there was a time when the hunt didn't go well or the winter lasted longer than expected and there was no food, our bodies needed a mechanism to survive— not just to stay alive for the moment but to assure long-term survival. If food was scarce then we needed both mental acuity to figure out where to get food and the physical energy to go get it. The body's ability to use its own stored body fat to convert into ketones and use as energy is the backup system during these times.

The overview of the science history: In 1911, Parisian physicians Gulep and Marie Bregan began documenting successfully treating epileptic children with fasting. This philosophy was most famously spread in the United States by Bernarr Macfadden, who was a physical fitness guru and publisher of a widely read health magazine, *Physical Culture*, for which circulation had reached 500,000 by the end of WWI. Macfadden claimed that fasting for three days to three weeks could alleviate and cure just about any disease, including epilepsy.

In 1921, Dr. Russell Wilder at the Mayo Clinic proposed that a ketogenic diet (KD) be tried in a series of pediatric patients with epilepsy. He correctly predicted that a ketone-producing dietary approach would be as effective as fasting and could be maintained for a much longer period of time. Wilder coined the term "ketogenic diet."

After the development of anticonvulsant therapy drugs, doctors began relying on a ketogenic diet much less frequently, but still reach for this diet as either the auxiliary treatment or the main course of action in the less severe cases in the number of patients who don't react well to the medication.

And there were challenges. The adherence rate for the ketogenic diet was low because families with children following this plan had a hard time incorporating it into their lifestyle. In an effort to make the ketogenic diet more palatable, Dr. Peter Huttenlocher, at the University of Chicago, in 1971 introduced a medium-chain triglyceride oil diet and suggested a reduction in fat intake from 80 percent to 65 percent, allowing less restriction of other foods.

A Brief Historical Snapshot of the Use of Ketogenic Eating

1900s: Ketones discovered in the urine of diabetics.

1920s: Used for drug-resistant epilepsy by Russell Wilder, MD, of the Mayo Clinic.

1967: Scientists discovered that ketones can replace glucose in the brain. Further research found that the brain runs 25 percent better on ketones than glucose.

1971: A diet composed of 60 percent MCT oil was shown more practical and just as successful for patients and their families. This modified macronutrient ratio allowed parents to create meal plans that the whole family could eat, making it more practical and sustainable.

1990s: Researchers found the keto diet to be effective for several rare neurological diseases.

2000s: Today, stars, athletes, CEOs, and regular people like us use the keto diet for weight loss and enhanced performance and brain function. It's been reported that Gwyneth Paltrow, LeBron James, Kim Kardashian, Halle Berry, Kobe Bryant, Tim Ferriss, and Ben Greenfield all follow a ketogenic lifestyle, and it's their preferred way to prepare their bodies when they need to perform at their peak.

The Evolution of the Keto Diet

So the big question is how did keto go from epilepsy, cancer, and dementia to brain function productivity and weight loss? During the 1950s and 1960s, researchers began to look at the ketogenic diet and its benefits to other aspects of health and its usefulness on various demographics from dementia patients to obese individuals—and the benefits kept multiplying.

The popularity of keto exploded around weight loss because it's so effective. It's effectiveness is a result of the physiological response of the body when reducing carbohydrates. On a keto plan, your insulin (the fat-storing hormone) levels drop greatly, which turns your body into a fat-burning machine. Insulin is the main catalyst for the hormonal domino effect that creates weight, but not just weight loss—literal fat loss. The lowering of insulin signals the increase of the mother of all fat-burning hormones in the body: human growth hormone (HGH). The increase in HGH has been shown not only to increase lipolysis but also maintain and build muscle at the same time, making it easier to lose the weight AND keep it off. HGH and insulin are opposites in function. HGH is focused on tissue repair, efficient fuel usage, and anti-inflammatory immune activity. Insulin is designed for energy storage, cellular division, and pro-inflammatory immune activity. A review in JAMA (*Journal of American Medical Associates*) looked at thirteen randomized control studies that showed people who lost weight using the keto diet lost MORE weight and were also able to keep more of it off than those on low-fat diets.

Keto Nutrition

Macro and Micronutrients

The human body must have nutrients for growth, energy, and other body functions. Two types of nutrients are required for the human body to both survive and thrive: micronutrients and macronutrients. All nutrients are essential to optimal health as each has a specific role in the body. Understanding how we get them, how they are used, and how much we need is essential.

Micronutrients

Micronutrients are nutrients required in a small portion (hence the prefix "micro") which maintain tissue and cell function and prevent disease and dysfunction. They include vitamins and minerals. Vitamins are necessary for energy production, immune function, blood clotting, cellular function, and physical and mental well-being. They are organic compounds made by animals and plants, and can be broken down by air, heat, or acid, such as vitamin C contained in oranges or iron contained in animal organ meat. Minerals, on the other hand, play an important role in growth, bone health, fluid balance, and keeping your muscles, heart, and brain working properly. They are inorganic compounds that exist in soil or water and cannot be broken down, such as sodium found in salt. The body maintains a very tight balance of both the inflow and outflow of micronutrients. The human body cannot produce vitamins and minerals, for the most part, and we must consume them from our food.

Vitamins and minerals can be divided into four categories:

> **Water-soluble Vitamins**: Vitamins that dissolve in water and are not stored in the body; they include vitamin C and all of the vitamin B complex (B1-thiamin, B2-riboflavin, B3-niacin, B5, B6, B12, biotin, folic acid).

Fat-soluble Vitamins: Vitamins that are absorbed along with fats and oils and can be stored in the body's fatty tissue: They include vitamins A, D, E, and K.

Macrominerals: You need larger amounts of macrominerals. They include calcium, phosphorus, magnesium, sodium, potassium, chloride, and sulfur.

Trace Minerals: You only need small amounts of trace minerals. They include iron, manganese, copper, iodine, zinc, cobalt, fluoride, and selenium.

Regardless of type, vitamins and minerals are absorbed in similar ways in your body and interact in many processes.

Micronutrients are often the topic of debate when discussing a switch to a ketogenic lifestyle. Many people believe cutting a specific food group, like fruits and grains, from your diet can lead to vitamin and mineral deficiencies. However, just as a person who removes animal protein from their diet can strategically consume various sources of plant proteins to compensate for animal protein, a well-formulated ketogenic diet can easily contain all micronutrients required for health. There is no vitamin or mineral contained in fruit or grain that is not contained in various vegetables, dairy, or animal protein. For example, bananas are touted for their potassium content, containing 422 mg, yet one cup of cooked swiss chard provides 961 mg of potassium, one-half of an avocado contains 487 mg of potassium, and one cup (156 grams) of frozen spinach contains 540 mg of potassium with far less sugar to accompany it.

It's important that we get a variety of foods in our diets to assure we are getting an adequate amount of all micronutrients. Below are some sources of micronutrients in foods.

Vitamins

Vitamin A (retinol)	Liver, dairy, fish; carotenoids (sweet potatoes, carrots, spinach)
Vitamin B1 (thiamine)	Whole grains, meat, fish
Vitamin B2 (riboflavin)	Organ meats, eggs, milk
Vitamin B3 (niacin)	Meat, salmon, leafy greens, beans
Vitamin B5 (pantothenic acid)	Organ meats, mushrooms, tuna, avocado
Vitamin B6 (pyridoxine)	Fish, milk, carrots, potatoes
Vitamin B7 (biotin)	Eggs, almonds, spinach, sweet potatoes
Vitamin B9 (folate)	Beef, liver, black-eyed peas, spinach, asparagus
Vitamin B12 (cobalamin)	Clams, fish, meat
Vitamin C (ascorbic acid)	Citrus fruits, bell peppers, Brussels sprouts
Vitamin D	Sunlight, fish oil, milk
Vitamin E	Sunflower seeds, wheat germ, almonds
Vitamin K	Leafy greens, soybeans, pumpkin

Minerals

Calcium:	Milk products, leafy greens, broccoli
Chloride:	Seaweed, salt, celery
Magnesium:	Almonds, cashews
Phosphorus:	Salmon, yogurt, turkey
Potassium:	Chard, spinach, avocados
Sodium:	Salt, beets, celery, chard
Sulfur:	Garlic, onions, Brussels sprouts, eggs, mineral water
Iron:	Shellfish, spinach, organ meat
Manganese:	pecans, peanuts
Copper:	Liver, crab, cashews

Zinc:	Oysters, crab, chickpeas
Iodine:	Seaweed, cod, yogurt
Fluoride:	Black tea, Kombucha, water, crab
Selenium:	Brazil nuts, sardines

Micronutrients are part of nearly every process in your body, and consuming an adequate amount of different vitamins and minerals is key to maintaining optimal health and may even help fight disease.

Macronutrients

According to the World Health Organization, there are three **main** macronutrients: carbohydrates, proteins, fats, and a bonus fourth—water. Macronutrients are used to give us energy—help us grow, repair, and develop. They each have their own role and functions in the body.

Carbohydrates

Carbohydrates are made up of chains of starch and sugar that the body breaks down into glucose. For most people glucose is the body's main source of energy. Because the body and brain require a constant sources of energy, the body is very efficient at storing glucose so it can have access to its primary source of energy even when you are not consuming food. Glucose is stored in the form of glycogen in the liver and muscles.

Think of carbohydrates as the fuel in a car or electricity in the house. They provide the energy to deliver the nutrients where they need to go. The purpose of a ketogenic diet is to convert the body from using carbohydrates as fuel to using ketones derived from fat.

Sources of carbohydrates:

- Whole grains (brown and wild rice, oats, amaranth, whole wheat)
- Starchy vegetables (potatoes, sweet potatoes, corn, beets)

- Legumes (beans, lentils, chickpeas, peas)
- Fruits (apple, oranges, berries, pears, bananas)

Because our body has the ability to create an alternate source of fuel for energy, as we will discuss in the next chapter, carbohydrates are not universally essential for a healthy diet.

Protein

Protein in the body is used beyond just muscle; in fact 16 percent of your body weight comes from protein alone. It is the foundation of every cell, including organs, bones, hair, enzymes, and all tissue, and is a core component to healthy immune function.

Protein provides amino acids, which are the building blocks of cell and muscle structure. In total, there are twenty types of amino acids, nine of which are essential—meaning that your body requires them from food—and eleven that are "nonessential" to the human diet because they can be made by the body.

Protein sources that contain all essential amino acids are considered "complete proteins." Complete proteins are often animal-based foods such as poultry, beef, veal, lamb, eggs, milk, yogurt, cheese, but also soymilk, tofu, edamame, and veggie burgers made from soy and quinoa.

Protein sources that do not contain all essential amino acids are considered "incomplete proteins." As a general rule grains (with the exception of quinoa), cereals, nuts, seeds, dried beans (with the exception of edamame, i.e., soy), dried peas, lentils, peanuts, and peanut butter do not contain all essential amino acids and are considered "incomplete" proteins. To get an adequate amount of protein on a plant-based diet, one would have to intentionally consume particular combinations of plant-based foods to create a complete amino acid profile. For example, many grains are deficient in the essential amino acid lysine, a nutrient found in beans. Conversely, many beans contain only small amounts of methionine, an amino acid found in larger supply in grains. When you consume both, they create a complementary protein source which becomes a complete protein. Of course this is just an informational example because for our purpose this would not be included in a ketogenic plan; one serving of either has more carbohydrates than a ketogenic plan can consume in an entire day.

The body has the ability to create energy (glucose) from protein in absence of carbohydrates. It's not its preferred source of fuel because it requires more metabolic work.

In general the amount of protein you need depends on various factors, including activity level, health and fitness goals, and age. A marathon runner or a bodybuilder needs three times the protein than someone going to a gym to lose a couple of pounds.

One way to determine if a food is a protein is to remember that a protein is anything that had eyes, has eyes, or will have eyes. A steak "had" eyes, fish "have" eyes, and an egg "will have" eyes.

Sources of protein:

- Fish and seafood (salmon, tuna, white fish, shrimp, crab, oysters)
- Poultry (chicken and turkey)
- Lean and organic meat (beef, lamb, venison)
- Eggs
- Dairy (minimally processed cheese, unsweetened yogurt, and non-dairy alternatives)
- Tofu and soy products (minimally processed)

Fat

Fats have been villainized in the western diet but are an essential part of all healthy diets and can be an essential component to health in a ketogenic eating plan. Dietary fats are essential to give your body energy, build cells, and help your body absorb some nutrients and produce important hormones. Fat also supports many of your body's functions such as blood clotting, muscle movement, and brain health. In fact your brain is made of 60 percent fat.

In the absence of carbohydrates and limited proteins, fat can be converted into fuel for energy in the form of ketones. This is the crux of the ketogenic diet.

Types of dietary fats

There are four major dietary fats in the foods we eat:

1. **Saturated Fats:** These fats are usually solid at room temperature and are found in dairy foods such as butter, cream, full-fat milk, and cheese; meat such as fatty cuts of beef, and lamb and chicken (especially chicken skin); processed meats like salami; and some plant-derived products such as palm oil, coconut, coconut milk, cream, and cooking margarine.

2. **Trans Fats:** Trans fats are unsaturated fats that have been processed and as a result behave like saturated fats. They are found in oils that have been hydrogenated and partly hydrogenated oils.

3. **Monounsaturated Fats:** Monounsaturated fats are found in olive and canola oil, avocados, and some nuts such as cashews and almonds.

4. **Polyunsaturated Fats:** Omega-3 fats are found in fish–especially oily fish; omega-6 fats are found in some oils such as safflower and soybean oil along with some nuts, including Brazil nuts.

A healthy ketogenic plan includes a variety of fats, while eliminating or at least minimizing trans fats.

Sources of fat:

- Full-fat dairy and organic, grass-fed butter
- Avocado and avocado oil
- Olives and olive oil
- Nuts (almonds, walnuts, cashews)
- Seeds (chia, pumpkin, flax)

- Fatty fish (salmon or trout)
- Animal meats
- Coconut oil

Ketogenic Macronutrient Ratio

A well-formulated ketogenic diet typically reduces total carbohydrate intake to less than 20 percent of your total daily caloric need. This is often referred to as between 20 and 50 grams per day. General ketogenic plans, including the mR40 method, suggest an average of 70 percent fat from total daily calories, 10 percent carbohydrate, and 20 percent protein. This roughly translates to about 165 grams fat, 40 grams carbohydrate, and 75 grams protein for a 2,000-calorie diet.

Examples of macronutrient breakdown of a ketogenic eating plan

Medicinal Ketosis (Used in research studies to treat epilepsy, cancer, dementia, Parkinson's, and other life-altering illnesses)

Fat 90 percent	Protein 10 percent
	Carbohydrates 0 percent

Fat 85 percent	Protein 15 percent
	Carbohydrates 0 percent

Nutritional Ketosis (Used for weight loss and health-boosting benefits)

Fat 80 percent	Protein 20 percent
	Carbohydrates 10 percent

Fat 75 percent	Protein 15 percent
	Carbohydrates 15 percent

Fat 75 percent	Protein 15 percent
	Carbohydrates 15 percent

Fat 60 percent	Protein 20 percent
	Carbohydrates 20 percent (beneficial for athletic performance)

Low Carb (NOT ketogenic) Can be beneficial for weight loss

Above 20 percent carbohydrates regardless of the percentage of fat and protein.

It's important that the protein amount on the ketogenic diet is kept moderate in comparison with other low-carb diets because eating too much protein can prevent ketosis. The amino acids in protein can be converted to glucose, so a ketogenic diet dictates consuming enough protein to preserve lean body mass, but will still cause ketosis.

Carb Tracking on a Ketogenic Plan

The main key to getting into ketosis is limiting the amount of carbohydrates you take in each day. By being familiar with what foods have higher amounts of carbohydrates and focusing on the ones with little to no carbs, most people will automatically stay within an acceptable carb intake range. However, if you are unsure or need an actual number, there are a couple of ways to go about it.

Total Carbs: Count the total amount of carbs in the food, regardless of the source of the carbohydrate. This is the easiest and safest way to assure you keep your carb intake low, especially for beginners.

Net Carbs: Net carbs are total carbs minus fiber and sugar alcohols, neither of which are absorbed by the body and have no effect on insulin levels. This type of carb totaling takes a bit more calculation and is most helpful in phase II of the program when you are familiar with your individual carb tolerance and give yourself more latitude of sweetener substitutes and higher fiber foods.

These average daily intake levels assume that you are also getting sufficient protein and healthy fats, and are doing some amount of daily activity. The ranges in each zone account for individual metabolic differences.

0-50 grams Total Carbs / 0-20 Net Carbs per day: Rapid Fat Loss Zone—Excellent way to produce rapid fat loss results. The lower end of the scale is not recommended for prolonged periods with the exception of achieving medicinal ketosis with medical supervision.

50-100 grams Total Carbs / 20-40 Net Carbs per day: Consistent Weight Loss Zone—Allows for steady drops in excess body fat and minimizing insulin production. Staying in this zone can create a consistent average weight loss of two-plus pounds a week.

100-150 grams Total Carbs / 40-60 Net Carbs per day: Maintenance Zone—Once you've reached your goal weight or your ideal body fat percentage, you can maintain this level of carbohydrate consumption while enjoying a wider range of vegetables, low glycemic load fruits, and legumes.

150-300 grams Total Carbs / 60-120 Net Carbs a day: Weight Gain Zone—Most unsuccessful dieters who attempt to be "healthy eaters" end up here due to the frequent intake of grain products, including whole grain breads, pastas, cereals, rice, potatoes. Despite trying to "do the right thing" (minimize fat, cut calories), people can still gain weight in spite of their best efforts.

300+ grams Total Carbs / 120+ Net Carbs a day: Rapid Weight Gain Zone—The Standard American Diet (SAD), which leads to an increased risk for obesity, metabolic syndrome, and type 2 diabetes. With the exception of extreme athletes and ultra-marathon runners, most people will produce excessive insulin and store excessive fat over the years when carbohydrate intake is at this level.

Calorie Counting of a Ketogenic Plan

Some people ask if it's necessary to count calories. I don't recommend counting calories on the mR40 method plan because it's generally not necessary. Because of the resulting hormone regulation of a ketogenic plan, the body naturally regulates calorie intake without extra effort. In other words, when in ketosis you simply won't have cravings or the desire to overeat or binge on foods. The body's leptin and ghrelin levels naturally regulate calorie consumption and hunger.

What Does a mR40 Ketogenic Meal Look Like?

Traditional Breakfast
Pancakes, eggs, orange juice, and berries
Atkins Breakfast
2 Slices of bacon and 2 scrambled eggs
mR40 Method Breakfast
1 cup of cooked greens, 2 scrambled eggs, and ½ avocado

How to Tell If You Are in Ketosis

Most people will enter a light nutritional ketosis (between 0.5-1.0 mmol/L on the blood ketone meter) within two or three days. It typically takes two to three weeks to get into a stable and optimal ketosis of 1.5-3.0 mmol/L and consistent levels of nutritional ketosis for 90 to 120 days to become fat adapted.

The ketogenic diet is the only weight loss program where you can use objective measures to determine if it's working. Cutting carbs alone isn't the point of a ketogenic diet. Any level of cutting carbs will be helpful toward weight loss. But to get all the benefits of ketosis, you need to raise ketones in your blood and lower your insulin levels through a change in macronutrient consumption.

Physical Signs of Ketosis...or at Least Getting There

There are several things people experience that may be physical signs that the body is converting from glucose as its metabolic fuel to a fat metabolism.

Short-Term Fatigue: As your body adjusts to its new metabolic process, you may feel tired and fatigued for the first few days. You may need to pull back on the intensity of your workouts and make sure you are getting enough sleep at night.

Thirst: Some people report feeling thirstier than usual. This may be a result of the side effect of water loss. Be sure to drink plenty water to avoid dehydration.

"Fruity" Breath: Your body creates byproducts when it breaks down fat into energy, one of which is acetone. Acetone is one of three ketones that is eliminated through your breath and is described as a "fruity" smell. It will eventually fade away, but until then just brush more often.

Appetite Suppression: When insulin levels drop, so do ghrelin levels, which decreases your appetite. This makes it physically easier to stick to your eating plan and eliminate cravings.

Increased Focus and Energy: Once you have fully converted to using fat as fuel, you will find you have all-day energy and then some. And since your brain runs 25 percent better on ketones than glucose, you will be focused and have more mental clarity than before.

Weight Loss: This is the whole point, right? Being in ketosis is literally using your own excess body fat as fuel. You will begin to notice weight loss pretty quickly in the beginning, then a slower but consistent drop in the scale after.

How to Measure Ketones

There are three types of ketone bodies: acetone, acetoacetate, and beta-hydroxybutyrate (BHB). Each of these three can be objectively tested to determine if you are actually burning fat as metabolic fuel.

Urine Strip Test

A urine test is the most commonly used method to measure ketones because it is cheap and easy. When your body produces excess acetoacetate ketones, they are not stored as fat like glucose (a huge plus of the keto diet). Instead they are expelled in the urine. Urine strips test acetoacetate expelled and change color based on the amount of ketones in the urine.

However, there are a few problems with the accuracy of urine ketone testing.

Research shows that urine ketone testing is not very accurate for high ketone levels. So it may be helpful when you first start a ketogenic diet to let you know you are going in the right direction, but it is not very accurate once you are well into ketosis. As your body becomes fat adapted, it uses ketones more efficiently and expels less in the urine. So you can be in a higher level of ketosis and the strips give you a low reading.

If you are dehydrated or overhydrated even slightly, it can throw off the reading. Dehydration can concentrate your urine and make you think you have a higher ketone level than you actually have. This is the biggest margin of error that occurs for most people using urine strips.

Urine tests can be helpful in the beginning, but I wouldn't take them as fact.

Ketone Blood Meter

Blood ketone testing measures beta-hydroxybutyrate (BHB— technically not a ketone but rather a sub-product of acetoacetate that acts like a ketone in the body) ketone bodies. Measuring ketone levels in your bloodstream removes factors that can distort the results, such as how drinking water can dilute urine results. Your body highly regulates the blood composition and shouldn't be affected by factors such as hydration, food consumption, or becoming keto-adapted when you've been in ketosis for an extended period of time.

Blood ketone ranges and what they mean:

Under .5 mml: Non-ketogenic State

Not considered ketosis. Your body is still using glucose as fuel.

.5 - 1.5 mml: Nutritional Ketosis

Your body has converted into using fat as fuel. All the benefits of keto state present themselves—weight loss, focus, energy, etc.

1.5 - 3.0 mml: Optimum Fat-Burning Zone

Maximum Fat-Burning Mode. (Basically you're a fat-burning machine.) All benefits of ketosis are maximized, especially weight loss.

3.0 +: Starvation Ketosis

Does not increase or decrease fat burning. Can indicate insufficient caloric intake. It's NOT recommended you sustain this level.

NOTE: Blood testing is the most accurate way to test if you are in ketosis. The levels mentioned in this chapter DO NOT apply to urine (which isn't accurate) or breath tests. They are testing different elements than the blood, so the scale is different.

Breath Meter

The third way to determine if you are producing enough ketones to be in ketosis is by measuring the ketones in your breath. The ketones in your breath are not the same as the ketones measured in blood. In ketosis, your liver breaks down fat for fuel, creating acetone as a byproduct. Some of that acetone is then released through your breath as isopropyl alcohol. Breath ketones are a real-time indicator of using fat as fuel, which is a huge advantage compared to measuring urine or blood ketones.

Note: Determining ketones via Breathalyzer can be affected by several factors, including alcohol consumption and water intake.

What Is the Keto Flu?

The "keto flu" is a collection of symptoms some people may experience when they are becoming fat adapted. Each person adjusts to the ketogenic diet differently. Many never feel any of these symptoms, some may feel one or two, and a few may feel three or more symptoms of the keto flu. It's estimated that about 10 percent of people feel one or some of these symptoms when first starting a keto diet. The theory is those who are most carb-dependent or have insulin malfunctions (type 2 diabetics, women with polycystic ovary syndrome) often have a longer time transitioning. Those who experience adverse signs will feel one or more of these symptoms during the first week of a keto diet, especially days 3-5. Fortunately, it's temporary, and you'll soon feel fine again. In fact, you'll likely have more energy than before you started the diet.

The symptoms of keto flu:

- Fatigue
- Headache
- Irritability
- Difficulty focusing ("brain fog")
- Lack of motivation
- Dizziness
- Sugar cravings
- Nausea
- Muscle cramps

The number and intensity of these symptoms vary greatly from person to person. The most important thing to remember is to stay hydrated and replace lost electrolytes.

How to Minimize the Symptoms and Duration of the Keto Flu

You can decrease the symptoms and the duration of the keto flu by doing several things to make your transition easier.

Stay Properly Hydrated

When you decrease glucose in your diet, it consequently decreases the amount of water your body holds. This happens because every glucose molecule has four water molecules attached to it. Staying hydrated can help with symptoms like fatigue and muscle cramping. Be sure to drink half your body weight in ounces of water every day and sixteen additional ounces for every hour of sweat-inducing exercises.

Increase Sodium

Ketogenic eating reduces glucose and decreases insulin levels. When your insulin levels drop, your body responds by excreting more sodium in the urine, along with water. Because of this, you'll probably find yourself urinating a lot more often in the first week or so of a keto diet. Since the loss of salt and water is responsible for most keto flu issues, increasing your intake of both can help reduce your symptoms significantly and often eliminate them altogether.

During the first few weeks of your keto transition, if you develop a headache, fatigue, nausea, dizziness, or other symptoms, drink a glass of water with half a teaspoon of salt stirred into it. This simple action may alleviate your keto flu symptoms within fifteen to thirty minutes. Feel free to do this twice a day or more, if needed. Adding a sprinkle of Himalayan sea salt to a daily half an avocado is a great way to keep sodium and potassium levels up as well. Other options are to create a soup with a bouillon cube or drink bone broth, chicken stock, or beef stock.

Increase Fat

When you've consumed plenty of water and made a conscious effort toward electrolyte balance, the next step is adding more fat. Consuming enough fat is an extremely important part of the adaptation of the keto diet. Consuming fat helps your body adapt to using its new fuel source. Unfortunately, years of western diet conditioning have convinced us that fat is bad. We have to unlearn what we have learned. Cook with and eat grass-fed butter. Use plenty of coconut oil and avocado oil; pour olive oil over your food, cook with it, and use it as dressing.

Is the Keto Flu the Same as Ketoacidosis?

No. The fear of ketoacidosis is often spread by people who do not understand how ketosis works. Although keto flu symptoms may seem intense and uncomfortable, this is not ketoacidosis. Ketoacidosis is when blood ketones reach harmful levels. Individuals with type 1 diabetes are at the highest risk of developing ketoacidosis and are not encouraged to do a keto diet unless specifically recommended and monitored by a medical professional. When ketogenic eating is done correctly, healthy individuals will typically produce enough insulin to prevent excessive ketones from forming, and blood levels of ketones should not reach a harmful level.

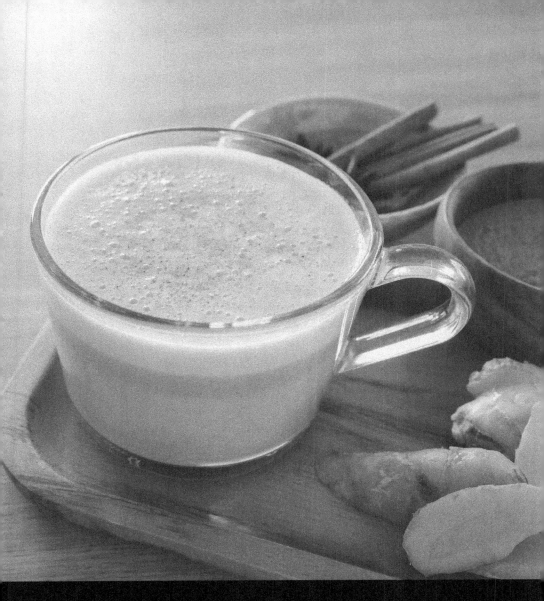

Chapter 5:

Fat Guards - Angiogenesis-
Inhibiting Foods

"For every disease He {God } has created a cure"

~ Holy Quran

The mR40 method is not saying, "It's not what you eat; it's how much you eat of it..." Nope, it's also what you eat. Science shows that many foods can prevent, halt, or even reverse heart disease, diabetes, obesity, cancer, and other life-threatening chronic diseases. The World Health Organization reports that 80 percent of cases of heart disease, stroke, and type 2 diabetes and 40 percent of all cancers are preventable. And I think everyone is well aware that 99 percent of obesity is completely preventable.

I have always believed that the food we eat either contributes to illness or contributes to health. And I became more intrigued with the idea of food as a means of healing after hearing a TED Talk by Dr. William Li, president and medical director of the Angiogenesis Foundation, who has conducted extensive research in angiogenesis-based medication and angiogenesis-inhibiting foods. At the time I was waiting for the result of a biopsy from a growth in my uterus, and in my effort to be prepared for whatever diagnosis was coming, my curious mind led me to the Internet and Li's TED Talk and subsequent research on angiogenesis-inhibiting foods. My biopsy came back benign, but my research had led me down a path that began to teach me more about nutrition and health on a cellular level.

What we eat and drink is enormously impactful when it comes to preventing disease. Over the past decade, the Angiogenesis Foundation has discovered and gathered evidence that fruits, vegetables, herbs, seafood, tea, coffee, and even chocolate contain natural bioactive substances that can prevent and intercept disease by influencing angiogenesis and other defense systems in the body.

The human body contains 60,000 miles of blood vessels, including 19 billion capillaries. It's helpful to think of blood vessels as rivers and capillaries as streams that flow off the rivers. Those capillaries deliver oxygen and nutrients to all the cells in our bodies. Angiogenesis is the development of new blood vessels (rivers). Through angiogenesis, the body has the ability to regulate the number of blood vessels that are present at any given time. It does this through an intricate system of checks and balances, stimulators and inhibitors of angiogenesis which are controlled by chemical signals within the body. These signals can stimulate the repair of broken blood vessels as well as create new blood vessels. In normal healthy adults, the rate of cell growth is balanced with the rate of cell death (apoptosis), so there is no excess tissue growth. The activity of angiogenesis is mostly suppressed to maintain this balance except for brief bursts during the female reproductive cycle in the regeneration of the endometrial lining of the uterus and corpus luteum formation during pregnancy for the development of the placenta, and wound healing.

The Health Affect?

If the body malfunctions and creates excess blood vessels, then problems like excess fat cells and even cancer can develop. When angiogenesis is off balance, it can contribute to a myriad of diseases. According to Li, "Insufficient angiogenesis—not enough blood vessels—leads to wounds that don't heal, heart attacks, legs without circulation, death from stroke, nerve damage. And on the other end, excessive angiogenesis—too many blood vessels—drives disease, and we see this in cancer, blindness, arthritis, obesity, and Alzheimer's disease."

According to the Angiogenesis Foundation, abnormal angiogenesis is the common denominator in more than seventy major diseases affecting more than a billion people worldwide that all look on the surface to be different from one another but share the same malfunction.

Angiogenesis-inhibiting compounds have been used to treat cancer for decades. It's fairly recently that researchers have begun to look to angiogenesis-inhibiting foods and compare their degree of effectiveness to cancer treatment drugs with the same goal. And like ketogenic eating, something discovered for a medical treatment has been found to be effective for weight loss.

I predict that angiogenesis-inhibiting compounds will be much like the ketogenic diet in the next five to ten years.

The ketogenic diet, too, began as a medical treatment, but its widespread health benefits became greater than the initial research suggested.

AI Fat Guards?

Fat cells are fed by blood vessels similar to how cancer cells are fed. Anti-angiogenic foods may normalize the growth of blood vessels to cells and in essence put your fat cells on a diet by regulating how they are fed. In otherwords that act as "Fat Guards" regulating the amount of fat that's stored. According to Li, in a study with obese mice given angiogenesis inhibitors, their weight decreased to a normal range, and when the inhibitors were stopped, their weight increased. With the reintroduction of the angiogenesis inhibitor, their weight dropped again and then increased again when the compound was stopped. From this and similar studies, we have learned that a constant supply of angiogenesis-inhibiting foods may be able to reduce weight and stave off obesity when consumed on a regular basis.

Of the many angiogenesis-inhibiting foods, the top ten that are considered "super angiogenesis inhibitors" and have been shown in research to work better than even some angiogenesis-inhibiting cancer drugs include...

AI Tea Combinations (Dragon Pearl, Jasmine, and Japanese Sencha)

Turmeric

Green Tea

Lavender

Citrus Fruits [Phase II of mR40 method]

Brassica Family of Vegetables (Cruciferous)

Red Grapes [Phase II of mR40 method]

Garlic

Soy

Berries [Phase II of mR40 method]

What makes these foods and other recommended foods in the mR40 method program so powerful is that the benefit of these same foods are intersectional with other health implications. In addition to being angiogenesis inhibitors, they are also anti-inflammatory, support the body's natural detoxification process, and encourage healing of the digestive tract. Each one of these health implications has significant impact on both our weight and our overall well-being. Remember, our goal with this program is not just weight loss but overall health.

AI Foods and Their Benefits

In this program I am putting an emphasis on the brassica family as your main source of vegetables in phase I. They are beneficial on multiple levels. In addition to their nutrient density of vitamins A and C, calcium, iron, vitamin B6, magnesium, potassium, and fiber, research shows that they prevent oxidative stress, induce detoxification enzymes, stimulate immune system, decrease the risk of cancers, inhibit malignant transformation and carcinogenic mutations, as well as reduce proliferation of cancer cells through their angiogenesis-inhibiting role.

Vegetables once referred to as the cruciferous family of vegetables are now being largely replaced by the Latin name *brassicaceae*. (In Latin, the word "brassica" simply translates as "cabbage," and cabbage is definitely a featured member of this vegetable group.)

The health benefits of this particular group of the brassica family cannot be understated.

In phase I of the program, recommended vegetables and limited fruits are based on two things: foods that have both the greatest angiogenesis-inhibiting qualities and are lowest on the glycemic load index, creating the least amount of insulin response. That means that although oranges are an angiogenesis-inhibiting food, they're reserved for phase II of your program when a slight increase in carbohydrates would not be of much consequence.

Brassica Family of Vegetables (Cruciferous)

Arugula (salad rocket)

Bok choy (pak-choi)

Broccoflower

Broccoli

Broccoli rabe (rapini)

Brussels sprouts

Cauliflower

Chinese broccoli (gai-lan)

Chinese cabbage or Napa cabbage

Collard greens

Daikon radish

Garden cress

Horseradish

Kale

Kohlrabi (German turnip)

Komatsuna (Japanese mustard spinach)

Mizuna (Japanese mustard)

Radish

Red cabbage

Romanesco

Savoy cabbage

Tatsoi (spinach mustard, rosette bok choy)

Turnip

Wasabi

Watercress

White cabbage

Wild broccoli

In phase II of the program, you will be able to incorporate citrus fruits, grapes, and berries due to their low glycemic load, further increasing your daily variety of AI foods. AI foods should be consumed on a consistent basis to benefit from weight management effects.

Citrus Fruits

Grapefruit: white, ruby red, oroblanco

Lemons: Meyer, eureka

Limes: key lime, Persian, kaffir

Mandarins: clementine, tangerine, tangelo, calamondin

Sweet oranges: blood orange, kumquat, navel, cara cara

Other kinds: citron, yuzu, ugli, Rangpur, pomelo, Buddha's hand, kinnow

One of the huge health benefits of being in a ketogenic state is its ability to reduce inflammation. Inflammation has detrimental effects on our health in a myriad of ways. We know that chronic inflammation can be associated with poor diets, environmental stress, and sedentary lifestyle, causing a variety of ailments such as:

- Heart disease
- Diabetes
- Arthritis
- Depression
- Crohn's disease
- Digestive disorders
- Anger disorders and aggressive behaviors
- And many other diseases and symptoms

Food choices and movement can have a beneficial effect in reducing chronic inflammation, offering both relief and prevention of many conditions connected with it. For example, omega-3 fatty acids have amazing anti-inflammatory properties that protect the body against the possible damage caused by inflammation on a cellular level. Omega-3 fatty acids interrupt the cycle of inflammation by inhibiting an enzyme that produces prostaglandins, which triggers inflammation.

Incorporating cold-water fish like salmon, herring, tuna, and mackerel—all of which you will find in the mR40 method program—can make a huge impact on the amount of inflammation in your body by giving you a diet rich in omega-3 fatty acids.

The complete list for the Angiogenesis Foundation foods includes a large variety of vegetables, fruits, oils, herbs, and even sweets. The mR40 method program includes many of these health-promoting foods in phases to achieve the best weight loss and health benefits.

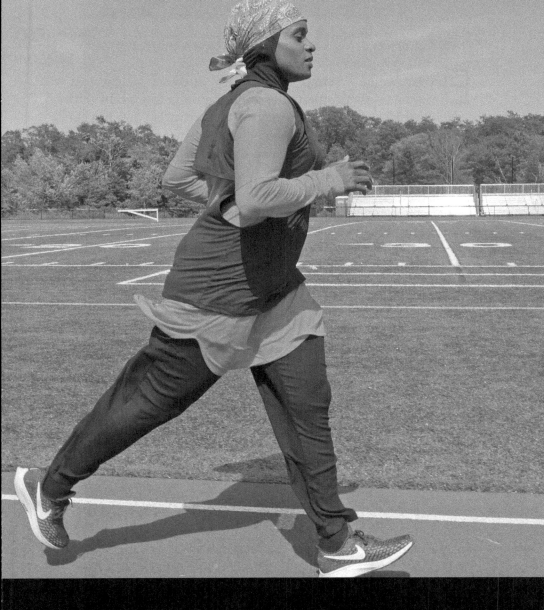

Chapter 6:

Move ... Faster

Exercise is an essential part of any effective weight loss program. Most people understand the need to exercise but underestimate the benefit exercise can provide, not just in weight loss but health. Movement is medicine, and that's not just a cliché. Just as medicine can both treat and cure disease, movement can do the same.

In many ways exercise is the "necessary evil" of modern times. For those of us living in developed nations, we no longer have to walk three miles—or even three minutes—just to get water. We have the convenience of simply walking into the next room in our houses. Our ancestors didn't need a weekly Zumba class, because simply doing daily chores required so much energy it was enough activity to keep them healthy.

But for us exercise is not cleaning the house and doing chores. Exercise is not taking care of your children, even if you have a rambunctious toddler. If these things were exercise, then obesity would not exist among women, since 87 percent of women above the age of twenty-one have one or more children. And until you move to the country, walk three miles to pump your water from a well every day, spend two hours harvesting your food, another four cooking it, and pee behind the bushes a half mile from your house, then you will need to engage in intentional movement, probably every day for the rest of your life.

It's great to go for a walk to get your blood flowing and maintain a healthy heart, but that's not good enough for most people who want to burn fat. The suggested goal of taking 10,000 steps a day was a campaign to get people to simply get up and move; it wasn't meant as a weight loss workout plan. It's true that doing resistance training as few as two days a week can literally reverse the early form of osteoporosis. And as few as thirty minutes of walking a day can get your body to metabolize glucose more efficiently and help you prevent diabetes. Very small changes in your everyday life can make a difference in your health. However, my goal is for the mR40 method to be transformative, so I'm suggesting you move with intention and intensity.

In this chapter you will learn how to minimize the time spent working out and maximize your results to create one of the most effective weight loss "hacks" possible. Just as all food is not the same, all exercise is not the same. But that's good news, because the benefits you will get will far outweigh the time investment.

Disclaimer: If you're new to exercise or have any preexisting condition, limitation, or disability, please check with your medical care provider before engaging in this or any other physical activity program.

History of High-Intensity Interval Training

If you've heard of Tabata training, then you've heard of the grandfather of all other modern high-intensity workouts. Tabata training is a form of high-intensity interval training (HIIT) discovered by Japanese scientist and head coach of the Japanese speed skating team Dr. Izumi Tabata and a team of researchers from the National Institute of Fitness and Sports in Tokyo in 1996.

They identified a range of health benefits with just twenty seconds' work at 170 percent of VO2 max and ten seconds of rest, repeated eight times (a total of four minutes). VO2 max is the volume (V) of oxygen (O2) that you consume while doing aerobic exercises like running and cycling. A higher VO2 max means that your body can take in more oxygen and deliver it to your muscles, enabling you to run or cycle faster for a given effort. Tabata's research proved that four minutes of this form of training can increase VO2 max by 28 percent compared to one hour of moderate-intensity cycling. Yes, four minutes of exercise exceeded the benefits of one hour.

When this news hit the mainstream fitness world, it caught like wildfire. And no wonder. This type of training spoke to our fast-paced lifestyle and desire for instant gratification. It promised to give quicker results in less time and significantly reduce the time people had to spend working out. It worked with every exercise modality. You could do Tabata cycling, running, lifting weights, or jumping rope. It didn't matter where a person's fitness level was, because it was based on individual rate of perceived exhaustion, so even beginners could do Tabata. But the problem was no one was truly doing the type of Tabata training done in the research. After all, even though we'd like to believe we are working at 170 percent of our maximum capacity, most of us aren't, and honestly probably can't due to the physiological and psychological stress that creates.

The second issue was that four minutes of exercise showed improvement in fitness level (VO2 max), not necessarily weight loss per se, especially for the general population who often engaged in exercise for the purpose of weight loss.

But all isn't lost, because in an effort to expand the application of Tabata training, subsequent studies have varied the time, intensity, and type of exercises done in various intervals (i.e., interval training), and the results are always better than steady state or moderate-intensity workouts. Not only does interval training result in you burning more fat over a longer period of time, like Tabata training, it increases your fitness level and strength quicker than any other type of workout. Consequently, you'll be able to do more physically, making your workouts much more effective toward your weight loss and fitness goals.

For clarity I am defining interval training as any exercise workout where you alternate between high intensity (7-10 on your rate of perceived exhaustion / 70 percent or higher of your HRM) and low intensity (2-5 on your rate of perceived exhaustion). These interval session are done in various time segments.

Not all interval training is Tabata training, but all Tabata training is interval training. Interval training can vary from doing fifteen minutes of high-intensity work with a ten-minute rest before repeating, or doing thirty seconds of high intensity with thirty seconds of rest and repeating.

The specific exercise is less important than the intensity in which you are working during the work portion. The "rest" or low-intensity portion of the workout will vary according to your fitness level and change as your body becomes more acclimated to this type of exercise. As shown in the original study of Tabata training and hundreds of studies after interval training increases VO2 max, in layman's terms that means your body will become more efficient at pumping blood through your body and you will need less rest time.

Get HIIT

Simply put, every benefit you are aware of that exercise provides, HIIT training multiplies it, while doing it in less time.

As explained previously, the metabolism is a complex chemical reaction in our body responsible for not just how we use and store fat but how our hormones interact and affect our health. HIIT training can literally change the way our metabolism does those things.

Drop More Weight Doing Less: HIIT training is the most effective way to not just burn fat but to build lean muscle and get fitter all at the same time. Dozens of studies have shown that people who perform high-intensity interval training seem to produce the same amount of weight loss doing twenty minutes of exercise as those who do sixty minutes of moderate-intensity exercise.

Become a Fat-Burning Machine: In addition to the number of calories you burn during your actual workout, your body continues to burn additional calories when you're done just to get back to normal resting state. This is called exercise post oxygen consumption, or EPOC for short. In the fitness marketing world, it's referred to as "afterburn." This afterburn taps into fat stores and continues to burn calories sometimes for hours after you've left the gym. Steady state exercise gives you a flow of afterburn that can last between two and four hours, but HIIT training can flood your EPOC for up to twenty-four hours. The more intense the workout, the longer your metabolism will stay elevated, burning more calories throughout the day.

Target Belly Fat: "How to get rid of belly fat" results in over 49 million results on Google. Certainly "What can I do to get rid of my belly fat" has to be the most common question I get. It's true we are aesthetically obsessed with flat abs in western culture, but that concern isn't without warrant. Belly fat—technically called visceral fat—is alive. It is the only fat on our body that actually produces hormones and shows a direct correlation to developing both type 2 diabetes and heart disease.

Weight loss in general will reduce belly fat, but HIIT training specifically has been shown in studies to target visceral fat more than traditional steady state exercises. In one study, researchers divided eighteen overweight subjects into groups. One group did moderate-intensity exercise, one group did high-intensity workouts, and the last group did no exercise for twelve weeks. The participants underwent body composition testing before and after the study. Interestingly enough, although none of the groups lost weight or changed their BMI or overall body fat percent, the high-intensity group decreased visceral fat (i.e., belly fat) while the moderate-intensity and control groups did not.

Insulin Sensitivity: Throughout this book I have spoken at length about the domino hormone insulin, its connection to glucose, and how it affects a wide range of health conditions. Exercise—and specifically HIIT—literally changes how the body metabolizes glucose, improving how efficiently the body can both access and use glucose. Insulin sensitivity, which describes the ability of the body's cells to take up or metabolize glucose, typically increases during and after exercise. Researchers Kessler, Sisson, and Short found that insulin sensitivity can improve by 23 to 58 percent over the course of two to sixteen weeks of HIIT workout regimen.

Lowers Cholesterol: One of the most common concerns about eating keto is its effect on cholesterol and developing heart disease as a result. Although, as explained earlier, I don't subscribe to this concern around a well-formulated ketogenic diet, adding the other component of the mR40 method makes this even less of a concern. I do not believe diet and exercise can be either separate or one prioritized over the other in an effective health plan. They were meant to complement one another. The mR40 HIIT program further enhances the ketogenic lifestyle by not just incorporating exercise but using the specific type of exercise that research has proven to raise HDL and lower LDL levels and by engaging in HIIT training three days a week for as few as eight weeks.

Decreases Blood Pressure: According to the World Health Organization, high blood pressure is responsible for nearly 13 percent of the world's deaths, more than 7 million deaths a year. Indeed, increased blood pressure is an important risk factor for cardiovascular diseases (including stroke and coronary artery disease). Research has shown that twelve weeks of HIIT training three times a week not only reduces blood pressure more than moderate-intensity exercise and medicine, but it improves arterial stiffness—a major contributing factor to heart disease and stroke.

mR40 Method Workouts

The workouts for the mR40 method include HIIT training two to three days a week, and steady state exercise two to three days a week. Below is an example of what your fitness routine may look like.

> Minimum / Beginner Exercisers: 2 days HIIT / 2 days steady state/moderate

> Moderate / Exercise Enthusiasts: 3 days HIIT / 2 days steady state/moderate

> Maximum / Exercise Veterans: 3 days HIIT / 2-3 days steady state/moderate

Note that these recommendations are independent of which phase of the mR40 method you are on or your current fitness level. It's important to start where you are in your fitness level and keep your workout basic, especially if you've never done HIIT before.

Time: You will be working as hard as YOU can, no matter what your fitness level. This is not about lifting a certain amount of weight or doing a designated number of reps of each exercise.

Your muscles cannot count. They only know fatigue. The most important concept is to push yourself and compete against your most worthy competitor: YOU.

Instead of having a designated number to reach, you write down the number of reps you did in the allotted time and then try to beat that number the next set.

mR40 HIIT Workouts: High-intensity interval training. This type of training requires you to bring your heart rate up to a high level and then back down. This constant fluctuation of your heart rate (i.e., intensity level) has been shown to burn more calories than long, slow, steady state workouts (i.e., keeping your heart rate steady throughout your entire workout).

The drawback of the HIIT workout (from a trainer's point of view) is that it is a self- determined intensity. The only person who knows if you are pushing yourself to your full potential is you. But a good technique to self-monitor and self-motivate is to count your reps. For each exercise you do in your designated time, literally count them and push to maintain or exceed your previous count WITHOUT compromising your form or changing the method. For example, if you do your first set of pushups "military style" without knees touching the ground and then switch to knee pushups in your third set, you can't compare the number to the previous sets. Changing the placement of the knees changes the intensity of the exercise and the muscles being worked.

Secondly, don't compromise your form to get in more reps. This is the main way people hurt themselves and sabotage their own results. If you start off doing ninety-degree knee angle squats, don't reduce your depth to get more in. Go down the same depth every time. Keeping these two points in mind will allow you to get great results from an mR40 recommended workout.

Because this program is based on the MOST effective techniques for rapid fat loss, I'm gonna skip all the singing to the choir about how important exercise is.

HIIT stands for high-intensity interval training, and it is one of the best ways to retain muscle while losing fat. It's by no means a new technique, however. If you consider this method in the truest sense of its name, it all comes down to a form of interval training.

HIIT training is the best way to burn fat without compromising your muscle tissue. There have been studies which show that some activities requiring long endurance, such as aerobics for example, can cause the breakdown of muscle tissue. This isn't a good thing. HIIT training allows your body to metabolize the fat while keeping your muscles intact.

There are many aspects of HIIT and interval training that are quite similar. The main difference is the intensity of the activity. You're probably now asking yourself what interval training is. Don't worry, everything will be much clearer by the time we're done here today.

How to Do mR40 HIIT Training

HIIT uses different levels of intensity during the same workout. You would add a considerably higher intensity activity to your low-intensity workout session. This can be achieved in many ways, allowing you to change things around if you find things getting boring, or just want to do something different.

[As with any exercise, if you're new to it, you have to be sure to clear it with your physician first. You don't want to be following any exercise program he or she doesn't agree will help you.]

For the workouts I designed for this program, I use a simpler perceived exertion scale (RPE). Something a little more relatable in terms of how labored your breathing should be and the levels of effort you should be feeling.

mR40 RPE Levels of Perceived Exertion

Level 1: Watching TV

Level 2: Strolling, walking through the mall window shopping

Level 3: Walking through the mall to get to a specific store

Level 4: I'm making an effort but I feel good and can carry on a conversation.

Level 5: I'm moving with intention, walking to be on time to a doctor's appointment.

Level 6: Speed-walking because I'm late to a doctor's appointment and hope they still take me so I don't have to reschedule.

Level 7: Running through the airport. OMG! I can't miss this plane.

Level 8: I can grunt in response to a questions and cannot keep this pace for more than a few minutes.

Level 9: I am probably going to die. I can't do this for more than sixty seconds.

Level 10: This is my ghost talking because I probably died sometime during that last set.

Once you experience or imagine those levels, keep in mind that your goal during this program is for your high-intensity work to be between 7 and 10 on the mR40 RPE scale, and your low-intensity rest should be between 2 and 5. As you become more familiar with HIIT training and become more conditioned both physically and mentally, you can go from 7 RPE to 10 RPE and still smile after your workout is done.

Here are some examples of how you can include HIIT in your exercise routine, depending on whether or not you are a beginner, intermediate, or advanced level interval trainer. I'll be using running for my examples, but you can use this method with just about any exercise, both cardio and resistance training.

Level 1 (Beginners): A beginner interval training program can use any movement that you are comfortable doing in good form. Below is an example using walking and jogging as the exercise. You can begin with a one-minute walk, followed by a one-minute jog at your personal RPE, whatever level of intensity that is for you. As you progress, you can decrease the "rest" or low-intensity time and increase the work time or high intensity. You simply repeat this as many times as needed for twenty consecutive minutes. It's important that your body gets used to this type of activity, especially if you haven't been exercising regularly until now.

Always begin with a five- to ten-minute walk or dynamic stretching movements to get your blood flowing and your muscles loosened up before you start. I recommend doing HIIT training two to three days a week as part of your weight loss plan. Again, it doesn't matter if you are doing sprints during the work portion or doing squats; the goal is for the intensity to be 8-10 on your RPE scale.

Sample: Routine - 20 Minutes

Walk at a 3-5 mR40 RPE and Jog at 8-10 mR40 RPE

Week 1: Walk 1 work / 1 minute rest [Repeat 10 times]

Week 2: Work 50 seconds / Rest 1 minute 10 seconds [Repeat 10 times]

Week 3: Work 40 seconds / Rest 1 minute 20 seconds [Repeat 10 times]

Week 4: Work 30 seconds / Rest 1 minute 30 seconds [Repeat 10 times]

Week 5: Work 20 seconds / Rest 1 minute 40 seconds [Repeat 10 times]

Week 6: Work 10 seconds / Rest 1 minute 50 seconds [Repeat 10 times]

Week 7: Level 2 (intermediate level)

Level 2 (Intermediate)

Up until now, you have simply been conditioning yourself in preparation for your HIIT program or routine. This is where it starts to get challenging, but the results will be much different than what you have seen to date. From here on out you'll be working in 40/20 HIIT splits. In my experience this is a good in-between time for both intermediate and veteran exercisers.

If using resistance training or body weight calisthenics, I recommend you choose five different exercises and do the set of five three to four rounds.

Weeks 7-9: Work 40 seconds / Rest 1 minute 20 seconds

[Repeat 3 times]

Weeks 10-12: Work 40 seconds / Rest 1 minute 20 seconds

[Repeat 4 times]

A sample routine may look like this

1. Squats: Work 40 seconds

20 seconds Rest

2. High Knees: Work 40 seconds

20 seconds Rest

3. Lunges: Work 40 seconds

20 seconds Rest

4. Pushups: Work 40 seconds

20 seconds Rest

5. Sit-ups: Work 40 seconds

Rest for 2 minutes

Repeat

And there you have it. One of the best ways to retain muscle while losing fat, and you can do it just about anywhere. Grab a bike, find a track, use a Stairmaster...just about anything is going to work. Are you up for the challenge?

You can find additional resources and exercise suggestions at mR40method.com/bookresources

Hack Your Workout Results

Multi-muscle movements

Our body almost never uses one muscle at a time, so the most functional way to work out is to incorporate multi-muscle movements into your workouts. Not only does it give you strength that will translate into your everyday activities, but it will also burn more calories. It will give you more bang for your buck. So opt for dumbbells more than resistance training machines at the gym. Instead of simply doing a standing bicep curl, simultaneously do a squat and bicep curl together or a lunge and overhead shoulder press at the same time.

Find more suggestions, videos, and workouts at mR40method. com/bookresources

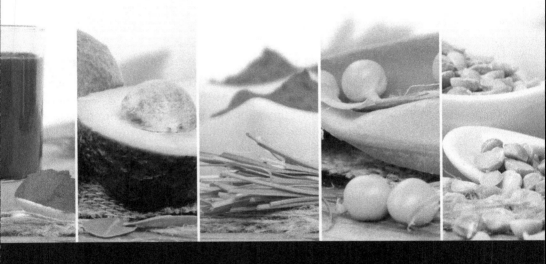

Chapter 7:

Putting It All Together

Now that you understand each concept of the mR40 method, let's put it all together to create a lifestyle of health and wellness. As mentioned earlier the mR40 method program is broken into two phases. Phase I is designed to strip your diet down to the basics and create rapid fat loss. Phase II gives more latitude in food choices and allows you more flexibility, making continued weight loss and weight maintenance sustainable. But more importantly it gives you elevated health and wellness. This is not a diet; it's a lifestyle.

Goal Setting

"Failing to plan is planning to fail"

When starting a new exercise program, most people fail or quit within the first four weeks. Statistics tell us 80 percent of people who make New Year's resolutions on January 1st quit pursuing them by February 1st without having achieved them. How many times have you promised yourself you would lose weight, eat healthier, or start exercising just to find yourself sitting in front of the TV, or scrolling Instagram, looking at fitness influencers, making yet another promise that you will start your journey again...tomorrow.

In my observation, most people fail at achieving their goals because they do not take the time to create a structured plan. My clients come to me, as a health and fitness coach, because I create the plan, I hold them accountable, and I help them see it through until they reach their goal.

You can achieve your goals in the same way, but it starts with setting clear goals. Before you begin any weight loss program or set any goal for that matter, it's important that you create a structured plan that's going to serve as a roadmap, guide, and motivation.

Define Your Goals, Motivation, and Commitment (Find Your Why)

Take some time to write down your goals. What do you want to accomplish? Why is that important to you? Set a realistic, clear, specific, and measurable long-term goal. In addition, create a few short-term interim goals to keep you on track for the long term. We have provided a worksheet on the next page to help you but also so you can share your goals with us and we can help hold you accountable.

Always set S.M.A.R.T. goals! Make each goal...

S - Specific

M - Measurable

A - Attainable

R - Relevant/rewarding

T - Time-bound/trackable

Further Goal-Setting Tips

State each goal as a positive statement. Be precise. Set priorities. WRITE GOALS DOWN.

Set performance goals, not outcome goals (set goals over which you have as much control as possible). For instance: "I will work out three times this week" instead of "I want to lose two pounds this week." The workout will lead to the weight loss. The weight loss does not lead to the workout.

Set realistic goals with realistic rewards.

You don't know where you are going unless you know where you've been. This could not be truer when it comes to fitness. Doing fitness assessments are important, not so you can compare yourself to others but rather so you will know how far you've come.

Do It the WRITE Way

Writing down how much weight you lifted or how many reps or sets you completed and how long it took to complete them gives you a record of your progress. It serves as encouragement when you need that extra reminder and it also serves as a way to see your consistency as you continue on your fitness journey.

You should write down every workout you do. If you use weights, write down how much, how many reps, and how many sets. If you are doing a bodyweight, write down how many reps and sets you are doing and how long it took you to do them.

Below is a template for your daily journal and a fitness tracker to write down your measurements, your workouts, and your diet.

Tracking Your Success

Get Naked

One great way to track your progress with your weight loss program is to take before and after photos. As much as you might hate the thought of getting your picture taken naked, the differences you will see can motivate you to even higher weight loss goals. And those "before" photos can be a huge wake-up call!

A study by the University of Alicante in Spain has shown that keeping a photo diary can keep dieters motivated, making them more likely to achieve their target weight. Photos serve as visual confirmation that all your hard work is paying off.

Strip down to nothing but your underwear. Take a full-length mirror selfie and save that image in your phone or computer. Remember that this whole exercise is for no one else but yourself. Don't share this picture with anyone, not even your spouse.

The reason you're doing this is not to look at yourself and feel depressed about how your body looks. Instead, treat yourself with the same love and compassion you give your partner. Would you cruelly point out how his stomach looks flabby or his arms aren't well toned?

Take pictures of yourself in your underwear at least every two weeks and compare them to your earlier pictures. Once you notice how your body is starting to look better after a few weeks of exercising, you will feel inspired and motivated to work out regularly!

How to take your photos

- Pick an uncluttered spot for your photo shoot, either in front of a wall or a door.
- Ladies, wear a sports bra and shorts or a bikini. You want to be able to see your waist, belly, thighs.
- Take the photo in portrait mode instead of landscape. You'll want to see yourself from head to toes, close enough to see some details.

- If you can get someone to take the shots, great! If not, use a timer—and a tripod, if you have one. I find ten seconds is just enough time to get into place.
- Look straight ahead and smile if you want. But don't cheat by sucking in your gut.

Take TWO SETS of pictures—one in your bra and underwear for your own motivation and one in clothes that you may or may not choose to share with me in a few weeks. I WOULD LOVE for you to share your photo journey with me; however, even if it's only for yourself, I still highly recommend you take photos. In fact I would say it's a required part of this program. Sometimes looking in the mirror on a daily basis does not allow us to see subtle changes.

Name:			Age:		Height:	

Date:	Week 1	Week 2	Week 3	Week 4	Week 5	Week 6
Weight						
BMI						
Body Fat %						
Body Muscle %						
Visceral Fat						
RMR						
Body Age						
Chest [Across Breast]						
Upper Waist [Smallest Area]						
Lower Waist [Belly Button]						
Hips [Widest Point]						
Waist-to-Hip						
Pushups [60 Seconds]						
Chair Squat [60 Seconds]						
Plank [60 Seconds]						
(Optional) Fasting Blood Sugar						
(Optional) Blood Pressure						
(Optional) Cholesterol						
Energy Level [1-10]						
Mood [1-10]						
Sleep Quality [1-10]						
Stress Level [1-10]						

Affirmations_____

_____

_____

_____

_____

_____

Today's Schedule

6am _____

_____   **Top 3 for the day**

7am _____

_____   _____

8am _____

_____   _____

9am _____

_____   _____

10am _____

_____

11am _____

_____   **Keeping Track**

12pm _____   Energy Level [1-10] _____
                                     Hours of Sleep [0-12] _____
_____   Sleep Quality [0-10] _____
                                     Energy Level [0-10] _____
1pm _____   Stress Level [1-10] _____
                                     Vegetables [0-10 servings]_____
_____   Ounces of Water: _____

2pm _____

_____

3pm _____

_____

4pm _____

_____

5pm _____

_____   Today I am grateful for

6pm _____   1. _____

_____   _____

7pm _____   _____

_____   2. _____

8pm _____   _____

_____   _____

                                     3. _____

                                     _____

                                     _____

Brain Dump _____

_____

_____

_____

_____

_____

___/___/___

Today's Workout Goal:

Fasted Cardio:					
Warm up/ Flexibility:					
Exercise:	Set 1 reps	Set 2 reps	Set 3 reps	Set 4 reps	Set 5 reps
1)					
2)					
3)					
4)					
5)					
6)					
7)					
Cool Down/Flexibility					

Nutrition _____

_____

_____

_____

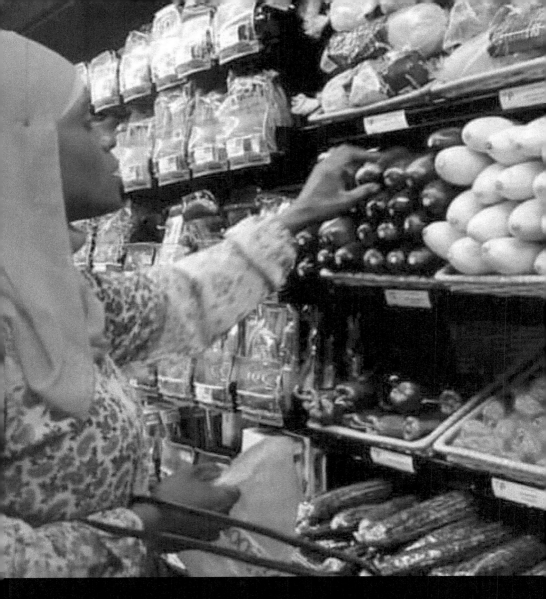

Chapter 8:

Lets Eat...NOT That!

Phase I

Phase I of the mR40 method requires you to strip your diet down to basic levels of simple whole foods, both to create simplicity in changing your eating habits as well as to supply your body with the very basics of nutrition from the most whole food choices. I encourage you to eat unpackaged and unprocessed foods. Avoid things that say "low fat" or "keto" or "paleo" approved. If there is room for these labels on the package, then it's probably processed in some way and should be avoided.

Intermittent fasting

During phase I you should be fasting sixteen to twenty hours every day. This fast should not be random but intentional and calculated into your daily eating plan. Determine a weekly fasting routine and stick to it. Don't fast just because you are running late and don't have time to eat. This haphazard eating routine will sabotage your mental discipline and preparedness.

What to Eat

Understanding the mR40 method will allow anyone to follow the program with success. If you do not live in the United States and don't have access to the same foods, you will still be able to apply the concepts and make substitutions with the foods you have access to with just a little research.

Phase I recommends...

#1 - Foods that have five grams or less of carbohydrates per serving

#2 - Foods and teas that are angiogenesis inhibiting

#3 – Foods that do not exceed twenty total grams of carbs per day

Fats

The main macronutrient needed is fat. Eating sufficient fat is essential in training your body to use fat as a source of fuel.

Examples: Olive Oil, Coconut Oil, Palm Oil, Cocoa Butter, Macadamia Nut Oil, Butter (Grass Fed), Ghee (Clarified Butter), Flaxseed Oil, Walnut Oil, Sesame Oil, Nut Oils, Avocado Oil

Meat and poultry

Animal protein is an important source of protein on the mR40 method diet, but you must remember to limit your protein to no more than 20 percent of your overall diet. This is NOT a high-protein diet.

Examples: Chicken, Beef, Venison, Lamb

Fish and seafood

Fish and seafood high in omega oils are encouraged as both a source of protein as well as healthy fat.

Examples: Halibut, Salmon, Albacore Tuna

Vegetables

Choosing vegetables that support the body's natural fat-burning process are prioritized in this plan. Get the majority of your vegetables from the brassicaceae and allium families of vegetables. In addition these families of vegetables are antioxidant and decrease inflammation. Other vegetables on the master list of foods are allowed, but you should prioritize these vegetables.

Examples: [Brassicaceae Family] Arugula, Bok Choy, Broccoli, Brussels Sprouts, Cabbage, Cauliflower, Collard Greens, Kale, Turnips [Allium Family] Chives, Garlic, Leeks, Onions, Scallions, Shallots

Nuts and seeds

Nuts are allowed in moderation. They are one of our healing foods and a great way to get fiber and additional protein in your diet; however, it's easy to overdo, so be careful and limit your quantities.

Examples: Almonds, Brazil Nuts, Cashews, Peanuts, Sesame Seeds, Sunflower Seeds, Walnuts

Herbs and spices

All natural herbs and spices are allowed and encouraged on the mR40 method. Flavoring your foods with the spices of your choice helps you to enjoy the same ingredients in completely different ways.

Coffee and teas

Coffee and tea (both caffeinated and decaffeinated) are allowed but no added sugar or flavored creamers. While fasting you must only consume black coffee and tea without sugar substitutes. Green tea in particular is highly recommended as a fat-inhibiting anti-angiogenesis beverage.

Nut "flours" and meals

Flours and meals made from nuts and seeds are welcomed additions to the mR40 method. They can allow you more creative freedom in making foods that are somewhat familiar and convenient.

Examples: Almond Flour, Almond Meal, Coconut Flour, Ground Flax Meal, and Psyllium Husk

Tomatoes and avocados

Although fruit is not recommended in the plan, tomatoes and avocados are exceptions to the rule in limited quantity.

Dairy

All dairy foods and milk products, including yogurt, contain a natural sugar called lactose. The higher the lactose content, the higher the amount of carbs. During phase 1 choose the dairy products with the lowest amount of carbohydrates.

Hard and aged cheese are allowed in phase I because of their low carbohydrate content. The longer a cheese is aged, the lower its carbohydrate content will be. For example, blue cheese and cheddar cheese have around 0.4 grams of carbs per ounce, and Parmesan cheese has about 0.9 grams in the same serving size. Foods containing less than 1 gram of carbohydrates per serving are considered to be very low in carbs.

Examples: Parmesan, swiss, feta, and cheddar (full fat) and soft cheese like brie, Monterey jack, mozzarella, and bleu cheese (full fat) are allowed.

Full fat heavy cream and sour cream are allowed but avoid milk, yogurt, and other dairy that contains more than 5 grams of carbohydrates per serving, especially flavored and low-fat varieties.

What NOT to Eat...

Grains

All grains are eliminated on the mR40 method, including bread (made with grain or potato), potatoes, corn, quinoa, pasta, cereal, tortillas, grains, rice (even brown rice). In particular, stay away from processed white carbs like cakes, cookies, and chips.

Sweeteners

All types of sugar and sweeteners are strictly removed in phase I of your program. White sugar, brown sugar, honey, agave nectar, coconut sugar, and any other form of natural or artificial sweeteners including aspartame, saccharin, acesulfame potassium, neotame, and sucralose are forbidden. Some zero-calorie substitutes have been shown in studies to have an effect on raising insulin levels as well as disrupting gut bacteria and therefore are not allowed on the mR40 plan. In phase II of the method, once your sugar addiction has been cured, you can add stevia, monk fruit, and erythritol into your diet in limited portions.

Fruit

Most fruits, with the exception of tomatoes and avocados, are not allowed on the MR40 method phase I. Yes, that includes bananas, pineapples, grapes, apples, etc. Although these fruits contain a plethora of nutrients, they also contain lots of fruit sugar (fructose), which causes spikes in insulin levels. You can enjoy low-glycemic-load fruits in phase II of the program or wait until you've earned a "flex day" to indulge.

Soft and Liquid Dairy

Not all dairy is out on the mR40 plan. Avoid low-fat milks that contain 0-2 percent of fat content, which is below the desired fat content. As fat content goes down, sugar (lactose) per serving goes up. Do not use evaporated or condensed milk, which are processed by evaporating some of their water content. Yes, this condenses the fat and protein but also condenses the lactose, which is natural sugar, that milk contains. Avoid milks and yogurts.

Non-Dairy Substitutes

Non-dairy substitutes like almond milk, soy milk, hemp milk, and coconut creamers are only allowed if they contain no other additives. Many store brands contain added sweeteners or thickeners made from ingredients that are not recommended on the mR40 list, so read ingredients carefully and make sure the carbohydrate content is less than five grams per serving. The best options of plain milk substitutes should only carry one to three grams of carbs per serving.

Processed Oils

Some oils have been shown to produce an inflammatory response and should be avoided. These include soybean oil, canola oil, corn oil, cottonseed oil, sunflower oil, peanut oil, sesame oil, and rice bran oil. Although the oils come from plants, they are overheated and processed using bleaches and chemical agents.

Alcohol

Do not drink alcohol of any kind. The human body cannot metabolize alcohol. It is in the most literal sense a toxin to the body Although many ketogenic plans indulge followers by allowing "low carb" alcoholic drinks, they do not account for the hormonal response alcohol has on the system, including the release of insulin and cortisol. This contradicts the homeostasis the mR40 method seeks to create.

Jump Start Your First Week

Sunday: Begin 24-hour fast

> 5:00 PM Stop eating

> Begin 24-hour fast

Monday: Continue 24-hour fast

> During the day: water, black coffee, black or green tea with no sugar

> Exercise: Do 90 minutes of steady state exercise while fasting to deplete glycogen muscle stores and accelerate ketosis.

> 5:00 PM Break fast

> Keto coffee / chai

Healing greens stir fry

2 to 3 ounces of protein of your choice

8:00 PM Stop eating

Tuesday: 20-hour fast

During the day: water, black coffee, black or green tea with no sugar

Exercise: Do 20- to 30-minute HIIT routine.

1:00 PM Break fast

Meal #1 includes

Keto coffee / chai

Meal of your choice

Optional snack in the day + A.I. tea

6:00 PM Meal #2

8:00 PM Stop eating

Wednesday: 16-hour fast

During the day: water, black coffee, black or green tea with no sugar

Exercise: 30 minutes of steady state exercise

Noon: Break fast

Meal #1 includes

Keto coffee / chai

Meal of your choice

Optional snack in the day + A.I. tea

6:00 PM Meal #2

8:00 PM Stop eating

Thursday: 16-hour fast

During the day: water, black coffee, black or green tea with no sugar

Exercise: Do 20- to 30-minute HIIT routine

Noon: Break fast

Meal #1 includes

Keto coffee / chai

Meal of your choice

Optional snack in the day + A.I. tea

6:00 PM Meal #2

8:00 PM Stop eating

Friday: 16-hour fast

During the day: water, black coffee, black or green tea with no sugar

Exercise: REST

Noon: Break fast

Meal #1 includes

Keto coffee / chai

Meal of your choice

Optional snack in the day + A.I. tea

6:00 PM Meal #2

8:00 PM Stop eating

Saturday: 16-hour fast

During the day: water, black coffee, black or green tea with no sugar

Exercise: Do 20- to 30-minute HIIT routine (optional long, slow cardio)

Noon: Break fast

Meal #1 includes

Keto coffee / chai

Meal of your choice

Optional snack in the day + A.I. tea

6:00 PM Meal #2

8:00 PM Stop eating

Sunday: 16-hour fast

> During the day: water, black coffee, black or green tea with no sugar

> Exercise: REST

> Noon: Break fast

> Meal #1 includes

> Keto coffee / chai

> Meal of your choice

> Optional snack in the day + A.I. tea

> 6:00 PM Meal #2

> 8:00 PM Stop eating

Phase II

Phase II on the mR40 method is EITHER after forty days OR when you have achieved your weight loss goals. By the end of phase I, you should have broken your sugar and carb addiction, reset your metabolism, and rebalanced your hormones. Now you can begin to incorporate angiogenesis-inhibiting fruits and low glycemic load foods into your long-term eating plan. Avoiding these things in phase I allowed you to enter ketosis easier and stay in ketosis longer.

Phase II is based on three things:

#1 – Foods that have ten grams or less of carbohydrates per serving or a glycemic load less than ten

#2 – A daily intake of foods and teas that are angiogenesis inhibiting

#3 – A limit of fifty total grams of carbs per day

When you begin to incorporate foods that contain more carbohydrates, it may take you out of ketosis more often than in phase I. The physiological goal of phase II is to be in "low grade" nutritional ketosis (.5-.75 mg blood ketones) during some part of each day. This can be achieved via intermittent fasting, increasing activity level, and/or keeping your carbohydrates lower.

As you expand the types of foods in your diet, be cognizant of how much you are consuming and how it affects your ketone levels. Each person is different based on both genetics and how long you have been fat adapted. The longer you are fat adapted, the more carbs you may be able to tolerate and the easier it will be for your body to transition in and out of a ketogenic state. You can do this by keeping track of the signs of being in ketosis or more accurately through blood or breath analysis.

If you are still trying to drop excess fat, anytime you hit a weight loss plateau remove phase II foods and return to phase I of the plan. This is called stripping—stripping your diet to the very basics of fat, protein, and dairy.

Intermittent fasting

In phase II of the mR40 method, I recommend two non-consecutive days of intermittent fasting of twenty to twenty-four hours. As in phase I, I do not recommend this be haphazard, but rather intentional and deliberate.

Research shows that intermittent fasting two non-consecutive days a week such as a Monday and a Thursday had more long-term adherence than either daily fasts or twenty-four-hour water fasts. Fasting twice a week entails limiting your caloric intake to 500 calories for women and 600 calories for men. This can be done with two small meals or one bigger meal after twenty hours of fasting.

Nutrition

*All Foods From Phase I

So, you are done with phase I of the mR40 method program and have reached your goal. Now what? The first question many people ask is if they will gain all the weight they lost just by looking at a french fry. The answer is no. As I have mentioned earlier, this is a lifestyle—not just a temporary diet.

We know that being in a state of ketosis has many health benefits, and it's not just about weight loss. Your healthy lifestyle goal is to get into ketosis at least a few hours each day or at minimum a couple of days a week.

Phase II of the mR40 method is our lifestyle method of the program. It's focused on maintaining weight loss, maintaining balanced insulin levels, and continuing to improve health, fitness, and well-being.

Focus on Low-Glycemic Load Foods

All calories are NOT created equal. What you eat and drink has long-term effects on your body and health but also an immediate effect on your body's rise in blood sugar and insulin levels. These fluctuations, which happen with every meal we eat, affect multiple aspects of your health as explained in the chapter on insulin. We've talked repeatedly in this book about the domino effect of insulin. Spikes and drops in insulin levels trigger a cascade of other hormonal, physiological and emotional changes.

This brings us to the glycemic index and the glycemic load, which are charts created from looking at the magnitude of that rise in blood sugar and help us understand how food impacts our bodies. The score indicates how food affects the rise in our insulin level when we consume it.

What is the Glycemic Index (GI)?

The glycemic index indicates how quickly foods break down into glucose (sugar) in your bloodstream. A food with a high GI raises blood sugar more than a food with a medium to low GI. A food which has a high GI will cause a large increase in blood sugar, while a food with a lower GI will not have much impact at all. The glycemic index uses a scale from 0 to 100, where 100 is pure glucose.

Foods with a GI of less than 55 are considered to have a low glycemic index, and thus will have smaller impact on blood sugar levels. Foods that fall in the mid-50s to mid-60s on the glycemic index chart are considered average, while a GI of 70 and above is considered high.

The problem with the glycemic index and why I didn't use it to qualify foods for phase II of the mR40 method is the fact that it standardizes each food to include fifty grams of carbohydrates, which leads to some peculiar distortions. For example, fifty grams of carbohydrates are both 2.8 ounces of a Snickers bar, which is about three-fourths of a king-size bar, or you can get fifty grams of carbohydrates in thirty-five ounces of pumpkin. It's hardly fair to compare the two when these portion sizes are so unrealistic! Like who only eat three-fourths of a Snickers?

What Is Glycemic Load (GL)?

The glycemic load, on the other hand, accounts for both portion and carbohydrates and is a better indicator of how a carbohydrate in the food will affect blood sugar. For our purposes of both balancing our insulin level and choosing food that minimizes the rise in blood sugar, the glycemic load is a better determiner of foods that best suit a healthy lifestyle.

Looking at the GL of foods also correctly places protein and fats in the category of preferred foods for a ketogenic diet. The GL scale is between 0 and 60. Generally, a GL of below 10 is considered low, 11 to 19 is considered moderate, and above 20 is considered high.

Because the GL of a food looks at both components, the same food can have a high GI but an overall low GL. For example, watermelon has a high GI of 72 because the standardized fifty grams used for the glycemic index count five cups of watermelon for a serving. Yet the standard serving size of one cup of watermelon has a low glycemic load of 7.2, which is more realistic for what the average person may eat in a sitting. The low GL indicates that a serving of watermelon won't have much impact on your blood sugar.

Carrots are another example of a low GL food that many people think will raise their blood sugar a lot—but it's not true. That's because carrots have a high GI of 71. However, what most people don't know is that the GL for carrots is only 6. Therefore, unless you're going to eat a pound and a half of carrots in one sitting, an average serving of carrots will have very little impact on blood glucose levels. That said, juicing carrots—which means consuming more carrots at once—will have a greater impact on blood glucose. The glycemic load of a carrot is 1 and the GL of eight ounces of carrot juice is 10.

The Method Behind The Madness

As a general rule all the foods in phase II of this program are foods that have a low glycemic load. (Not to be confused with the glycemic index of the food.) Remember, they are different and will present you with a different set of "acceptable" foods.

Sticking with foods that have a low glycemic load will allow you to maintain your weight loss. It also gives some latitude in the types of food you eat.

Foods in Phase II

Continue to enjoy all the foods in Phase 1 while adding the following

Sweeteners

Stevia, monk fruit, and erythritol are zero-calorie sugar substitutes that are allowed in phase II of the mR40 method. After completely eliminating added sweeteners for forty days, you should be completely cured of any sugar addiction you may have had. After this habit is broken, then you can begin to incorporate sugar substitutes into your coffee or tea and foods that do not raise insulin levels to your food and beverages. It's important that you break both the physiological addiction and psychological habit to sweeteners.

Monk Fruit

Monk fruit is an excellent sugar substitute for keto, paleo, and other low-carb baking recipes.

Monk fruit is 200 times sweeter than sugar, so very little is required in cooking.

Monk fruit has no carbs and does not spike insulin.

Monk fruit is generally free of side effects.

There's some suggestion that monk fruit may have anti-inflammatory benefits.

Stevia

Stevia has no impact on blood sugar.

Stevia contains magnesium, zinc, potassium, and vitamin B3.

Due to its sweetness, a lot less of it is required.

Erythritol

Erythritol occurs naturally in fruits and from fermentation.

Erythritol is a sugar alcohol.

Erythritol has zero bearing on blood sugar and no side effects unless eaten in large doses.

When erythritol is taken in large doses, nausea is the most common complaint.

Erythritol is very easy on the stomach and doesn't cause bloating or gas like some sweeteners do in higher amounts.

Low Glycemic Load Fruits

Most fruit is limited to your "flex day" on the mR40 method. However, in phase II you may consume fruits with a low glycemic load of 5 and under and paired with a protein. For example, you can have a quarter cup of blueberries with a serving of almonds as a snack in phase II. This comes with several ***asterisks***. Be very LIMITED in the amount of approved fruits you incorporate into your diet, because fruit contains sugar (fructose) and will affect both your insulin level and your ability to be in ketosis. Consume fruit no more than twice a week. And if your weight loss stops or if you show signs of being bumped out of ketosis, remove fruits first.

Secondly, we want to prioritize fruits with angiogenesis-inhibiting properties to maximize the health benefits and nutrients.

Examples of approved fruits (in order of glycemic load of 120g). Bolded letters indicate angiogenesis-inhibiting properties: Lime (1), **Strawberry (1)**, Fresh Apricot (3), **Fresh Cherries (3)** Grapefruit (3), Lemon (3), Watermelon (4), Cantaloupe (4), Guava (4), Nectarines (4), **Oranges (4),** Pear (4), Watermelon (4), **Fresh Blueberries (5),** Fresh Peaches (5), Fresh Plums (5)

Dairy [consume in moderation]:

You can now begin to add softer dairy products like plain Greek yogurt and unflavored kefir to your diet. BUT be very conscious that they have a much higher carbohydrate content. If weight loss stalls, this should be the first category of food you remove from your diet, because it can easily add too much sugar (in the form of lactose) and carbs to your diet. You should still avoid flavored and low-fat varieties of dairy.

Other Allowed Foods

Hummus. Hummus is another food that's allowed, but you'll want to be careful about servings. Although it contains less than two grams of carbs per tablespoon, it can be easy to go overboard.

Find a Comprehensive Food List in Chapter 11.

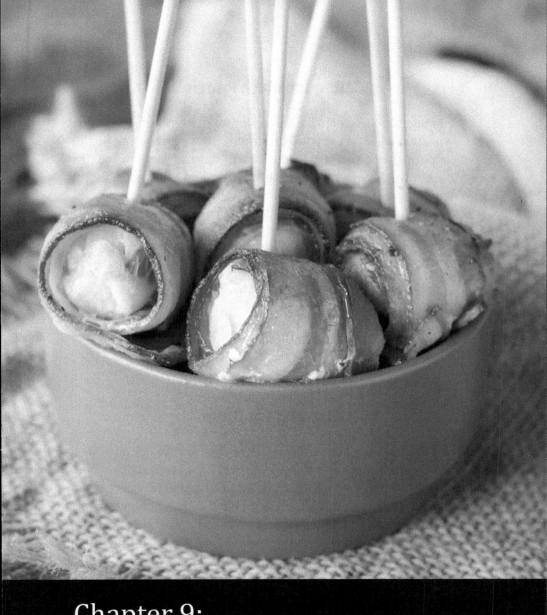

Chapter 9:

Eating Too Much Protein

A ketogenic diet is NOT a high-protein diet. In fact, too much protein will prevent you from entering a state of ketosis. In the absence of glucose from carbohydrates, your body will turn extra protein into glucose through a process called gluconeogenesis. When you are attempting to follow a ketogenic eating plan and more than about 20 percent of your diet comes from fat and less than 10 percent comes from carbohydrates, then your weight loss and weight loss experience have negative effects.

Fat loss is more likely to be temporary.

There is no cognitive improvement.

There is no anti-aging or cellular detox.

You may experience an energy roller coaster.

Snacking Too Often

Trying to combine diet methods is a recipe for disaster. The idea that you need to "graze" or eat three meals and two snacks does not apply to ketogenic eating. Usually when people feel the need to snack a lot on a keto plan, it's more a habit than actual hunger. The reduction in insulin as a result of lowering carbohydrates—reducing the frequency that you feel hungry—and a fat-adapted metabolism sustain energy much longer than a glucose-based metabolism. Don't snack for the sake of snacking. Pay attention to your hunger signals.

Eating "Low-Carb" Processed Foods

More and more people are discovering the benefits of low-carb and ketogenic eating. In January of 2019, even SlimFast came out with a "keto shake." Low carb products have become a billion-dollar industry, and within that are companies that are concerned about the capitalism, not the science. As a result the ingredients in "low-carb" foods aren't always low carb. Cauliflower pizza can have potato starch in it, or low-carb drinks are sweetened with insulin-raising xylitol. Remember, ketogenic eating is whole-food eating. It's safest to stay clear of foods in the box. If there's room to write "keto friendly" or "low-carb," then it's written on a package, which means it's probably processed in some way.

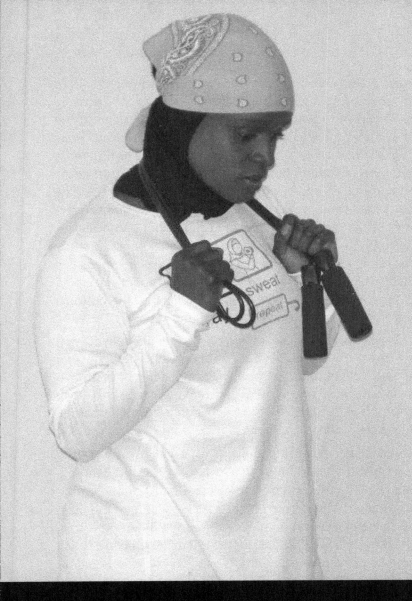

Chapter 10:

Hack Your Weight Loss Results

We are often encouraged to drink more water with little information about how beneficial staying hydrated actually is. When it comes to weight loss, water is probably one of the simplest ways to increase your metabolism and improve your results. We all know that water keeps you hydrated, a basic human need, but water also literally makes your metabolism run faster and burn more calories according to a German research study. The study found that drinking six cups of cold water a day (that's forty-eight ounces) can raise resting metabolism by about fifty calories daily—enough to shed five pounds in a year. Another study published in the *Journal of Clinical Endocrinology and Metabolism* found that within ten minutes of drinking water (about seventeen ounces), the metabolic rate increased by 30 percent in both men and women and lasted for thirty to forty minutes.

On the other hand it's also known that even mild dehydration will slow down the metabolism by as much as 3 percent. And that's just one effect of dehydration. Other studies have shown that just a 2 percent dehydration level can trigger short-term memory problems and difficulty focusing on a computer screen or printed page.

The idea that everyone should drink a gallon of water to be "fit and healthy" is a myth that was born in bodybuilding gyms. Many bodybuilders are known to carry gallon jugs of water around with them from one exercise machine to the next, chugging loads of water. When the non-bodybuilders saw this, they looked at muscles and flat abs and figured, *If I can't bench press three hundred pounds, then I can at least drink a gallon of water.* But the truth is a gallon of water a day is not necessary for most people. Bodybuilders in general have very low body fat and lots of lean muscle. There are several factors that require bodybuilders and those with a high percentage of body muscle to drink more water. Key among those reasons is the fact that muscles contain seven times as much water as fat does and require much more water to hydrate.

The goal is never to feel thirsty. When you actually feel your throat dry and you crave water, that's your body's warning system letting you know you are already dehydrated. Once you feel the signs of thirst, you may already be as much as 2 percent dehydrated.

Drink smaller portions throughout the day. The body only has the ability to absorb and use a maximum of twenty-four ounces of water every hour. Research done in marathon athletes found that sixteen to twenty-four fluid ounces per hour schedule during athletic events prevented dehydration. So when you sit down and drink a liter of water, you have to go to the bathroom because the body is expelling most of the unused liquid. To reduce urination frequency and become more efficient in your body's use of the water you are drinking, take in small portions of water throughout the day. Keep a water bottle nearby and drink a cup or two no more than every thirty minutes. This makes your hydration a much more effective metabolism-boosting habit.

Drink half your body weight in water a day: The idea that every person should drink sixty-four ounces of water a day is an urban myth of sorts. No one knows where that number came from, nor is it practical based on what we know about the difference in metabolism and energy expenditure based on body weight and size alone. A person who's 115 pounds does not need the same number of calories or nutrients as a person who's 300 pounds. Nor do they burn the same number of calories when engaged in any movement. So to assume that a 115-pound person and a 300-pound person should drink the same amount of water on a daily basis goes against reason.

The Amount of Water in the Body Depends on Many Factors:

Body size: Larger people have more physical mass and thus more body water and should compensate accordingly. In other words, someone who is 300 pounds will need more water than someone who is 150 pounds.

Body composition: The lower the percentage of body fat, the greater the percentage of water in the body. Skeletal muscle is about 72 to 73 percent water, while only about 10 percent of adipose tissue (fat) is water. So the leaner you are, the less water you have to maintain.

Gender: Males have more body water because they have more muscle mass. And as pointed out above, muscle has and requires seven times more water than fat tissue.

Age: We are born comprised of about 78 percent water and decrease to 55 percent by the time we reach old age. Younger people have more body water.

Activity Level: When engaging in exercise the average person needs to add eight ounces of water for every thirty minutes of exercise. Less for lighter weight and/or cooler temperatures and a little more for heavier individuals and/or hot temperatures.

Water is essential to sustain life. Less dramatic are the small effects dehydration can have on body functions and health.

Symptoms by percentage body weight water loss:[3]

Percent Water Loss	Symptoms
0 percent	none, optimal performance, normal heat regulation
1 percent	thirst stimulated, heat regulation during exercise altered, performance declines
2 percent	further decrease in heat regulation, hinders performance, increased thirst
3 percent	more of the same (worsening performance)
4 percent	exercise performance cut by 20 to 30 percent
5 percent	headache, irritability, "spaced-out" feeling, fatigue
6 percent	weakness, severe loss of thermoregulation
7 percent	collapse likely unless exercise stops
10 percent	comatose
11 percent	death likely

---

[3] Nutrition for Cyclists, Grandjean & Ruud, *Clinics in Sports Med.* Vol 13(1); 235-246. Jan 1994.

Drink water within thirty minutes of rising: During normal sleep the metabolic rate reduces by around 15 percent and reaches a minimum in the morning in an average circadian pattern (pattern of alertness and sleep). Several studies have proven that drinking water causes a metabolism boost, and drinking water upon rising is a great way to kick your metabolism into overdrive. Start each morning with sixteen ounces of water, and like participants in a 2007 study published in *The Journal of Clinical Endocrinology & Metabolism*, you will boost your metabolic rate 24 percent above normal for the first hour of your day.

Drink two cups (sixteen ounces) of water before every meal. In a twelve-week study that tracked water intake and weight loss, scientists from Virginia found subjects who drank two cups of water before each meal lost five pounds more than those who did not. Those who drank water before their meals lost an average of 15.5 pounds compared to those who did not and lost an average of eleven pounds during the study. If you do this three times daily—at breakfast, lunch, and dinner—you have already consumed forty-eight ounces of water. Add the sixteen ounces from when you woke up, and you are already at sixty ounces of water before bedtime.

Drink cold water. Drinking any water—cold or hot, carbonated or noncarbonated, distilled or spring, flavored with a teabag or a slice of lemon—has benefits, but drinking cold water is particularly beneficial for weight loss due to the thermogenic response of the body. When you drink cold water, your body increases energy expenditure (i.e., burns calories) to prevent your internal body temperature from dropping as a result of the water being colder than the body. So when you are at a restaurant, ask for a few pieces of ice in your complimentary water and keep your water bottle in the fridge when not in use, or better yet use a thermo-water jug that will keep your ice water cool.

Drink water before bed. This habit falls under the same philosophy as drinking water when you wake up in the morning. The body's metabolic rate drops while we are sleeping. In anticipation of this drop, drinking a couple of glasses of water before going to bed can keep your metabolism revving when it would otherwise have a 15 percent drop.

Sleep Away the Fat

One of the biggest regrets I have from my younger years, when I was growing my health and fitness business, is the lack of sleep I got. I thought it meant I was doing important things when I created a schedule that only allowed for three to four hours of sleep a night. Boy, was I dead wrong! I not only robbed my body of one of the most essential natural health benefits, but I also reduced my level of productivity, speed of thought, and worst of all set a bad example for my children, who now as young adults seem to think it's a badge of honor to be so busy, they only sleep three hours. It's an example that I am constantly trying to reverse.

Sleep is not meant to simply allow us to rest; it literally allows our body to heal from the inside out. It physically restores, rebuilds, regenerates cells, detoxes our brain, and resets our hormones to allow not just our mind but our body to function in an optimal state.

During sleep, you usually go through five stages of sleep. Simplified, stages 1-2 are light sleep, 3-4 deep sleep, and the fifth stage is REM sleep, also referred to as rapid eye movement sleep.

REM is arguably the most important of all the stages of sleep. You generally enter REM sleep about ninety minutes after initially falling asleep, and each REM stage can last up to an hour. An average adult has five to six REM cycles each night. REM sleep plays an important role in learning and memory function, since this is when your brain consolidates and processes information from the day before so that it can be stored in your long-term memory. When we fail to fall into REM sleep or get less of it, we lose the essential functions that happen during that stage of sleep.

The Lack Of Sleep Could Be Making You Fat

Remember pulling an all-nighter studying for a test in high school or college? Alongside those books and papers sat a bag of chips or cookies—"essential" studying snacks. Those extra munchies weren't brain food but the result of our body not getting enough sleep, and here's why. Sleep regulates several hormones responsible for both appetite and fat storage.

Leptin and Ghrelin

Those two "hunger hormones" we discussed earlier, leptin and ghrelin, are both directly affected by sleep, or the lack thereof. If we use an analogy of a train, leptin is the conductor in the front, pushing the gas, telling us to eat, and ghrelin is the conductor in the back of the train pulling the brake, telling us to stop. When you don't get enough sleep, you end up with too little leptin in your body, which makes your brain think you are hungry even when you aren't. This can lead to you constantly feeling hungry and eating more calories than you need. Even worse, low levels of leptin also signal your body to slow down your metabolism and store those calories as fat so you'll have enough energy the next time you need it. When ghrelin levels are up, our brain starts the series of signals that tell our stomach we are hungry and warn our body to slow down the metabolism and start storing fat "just in case" we don't have a meal coming. But when we don't get enough sleep, ghrelin levels stay elevated, slowing down our metabolism and increasing fat storage.

Cortisol and Insulin

Cortisol is called the "stress hormone" because it is secreted by the adrenal glands during times of fear or stress, whenever your body goes into the fight-or-flight response. Your body is designed to use short bursts of this hormone during acute stress; however, when cortisol levels are too high for too long, this hormone can hurt you more than it helps. Chronic high levels may contribute to not just inflammation as mentioned earlier but high blood pressure, depression, diabetes, and weight gain. Insomnia causes high cortisol for up to twenty-four hours. Cortisol is a trigger hormone for insulin, both of which turn on the fat storage switch. So not only does insufficient sleep increase your risk for disease, it increases your chance to gain weight and can prevent you from losing weight.

Cancer Soldiers

Our bodies have a natural mechanism for ridding our bodies of the first signs of many diseases. We have thousands of soldiers working in shifts to keep us healthy without us even knowing or feeling it. We even have an anti-cancer battalion of cells called TNF— tumor necrosis factor—that pump through our veins when we are asleep, seeking out potential cancer-causing cells and destroying them. But lack of sleeps decreases TNF cells. Research has shown that people who stayed up until 3 a.m. had one-third fewer cells containing TNF the next day, and that the effectiveness of those remaining was greatly reduced.

Tips on getting a better night's sleep

#1. Plan enough hours of sleep. The average adult needs between seven to nine hours of sleep a night as this will allow the major body systems to rest and the body's cells to be renewed. With the average American reporting 6.8 hours as opposed to nine hours a century ago, and around 30 percent of adults reporting sleeping less than six hours per night, we are a seriously sleep-deprived nation. To make matters worse research shows that women actually need more sleep than men and should aim for the longer hours, yet women are less likely than their male counterpart or their spouse to get more sleep. Not getting an adequate amount of sleep decreases the amount of REM sleep we experience, which is arguably the most important portion of our sleep cycle. It's during REM that our cells have the most rapid turnover rate, and our brain cleans out a toxic protein called beta-amyloid from brain tissue. Beta-amyloid is a sort of residual compound that develops from brain activity. Throughout the day when we are using our brain for everything from making critical decisions to remembering to brush our teeth, our brain is busy getting everything right and theoretically doesn't have time to multitask by detoxing and performing "alert brain" functions simultaneously. So sleep becomes a critical time for our brain to rid the body of this toxin. Excess beta-amyloid has been connected to "dirty brain" diseases like Alzheimer's that show a buildup of this toxin. Getting an adequate amount of sleep is a disease-preventive health habit.

Count backward to determine an appropriate bedtime. If you know you need to get up at 6:00 a.m. to start your day and you are planning for eight hours of sleep, then you need to be asleep by 10:00 p.m.

#2. Create a bedtime routine. When we were kids we had a bedtime routine every night. I knew when my mom asked about my homework, then instructed me to take a shower, that it was the beginning of the end of the day. I was not only consciously aware bed would soon follow, but my body also got subconscious signals. As adults our bodies' needs are similar but our habits change.

Our body is designed to create physiological responses from environmental clues. This is why you may feel joy when you taste cotton candy and recall a fond childhood memory associated with it. Or why someone who's afraid of clowns may feel anxious simply seeing a carnival, even if there is no actual clown in sight. Creating a regular bedtime routine, such as taking a warm shower and going to bed at the same time every night, can help to signal the body that it is time for rest, thereby making falling asleep at the desired time easier.

#3. Prepare your brain to rest. Our electronic gadgets have become such a huge part of our daily lives that it's often hard to put them down—even at bedtime. With surveys showing that 90 percent of American use electronics (TVs, tablets, smartphones, laptops, or other electronic devices) within one hour of going to bed and 60 percent of them fall asleep watching TV, it's no wonder the US Department of Health and Human Services reports 68 percent or roughly 164 million Americans struggle with sleep at least once a week, and two out of every ten Americans have a sleep disorder.

The blue light emitted by the screens of these devices restrain the production of melatonin, the hormone that controls your sleep/wake cycle, or the circadian rhythm of the brain that tells you to go to sleep. When you fall asleep watching TV, with your phone in your hand, or even reading your e-tablet, your quality of sleep will be significantly compromised. A study by researchers at Harvard Medical School found that compared to reading a paper book, people who read from an e-book needed an additional ten minutes to fall asleep. They experienced ninety minutes of delayed melatonin onset—and had half the amount of melatonin released. They also had diminished REM sleep. Over time, these effects can add up to a significant, chronic deficiency in sleep.

Try setting an electronics curfew before bed. The National Sleep Foundation recommends turning off all devices an hour prior to bedtime. Use the time to read a paper book or magazine, catch up with the day's events with your spouse, or just listen to music or an audiobook. Allowing your body to restore its natural circadian rhythm will improve the health benefits of your sleep.

#4. Keep a journal: Writing in a gratitude journal improves sleep, according to a 2011 study published in *Applied Psychology: Health and Well-Being*. Spend just fifteen minutes jotting down a few grateful sentiments before bed, and you may sleep better and longer. We will delve deeper into this in the subsequent chapter on gratitude.

Big Fat Worry Warts: Stress = Fat

There are certain universal truths, and the fact that stress is a part of life from the day we are born to the day we die is one of them. A baby is stressed when they are hungry or wet. The corporate professional facing a deadline for a project is stressed. The farmer in Africa is stressed when his cows are sick. The stay-at-home mom is stressed being overwhelmed with the pressures of being the perfect mom. The school kid feels stress when taking a test. No matter what our stage of life, where in the world we reside, or what our socioeconomic status is, we all feel stress on a daily basis.

"Life is 10 percent what happens to you
and 90 percent of how you respond to it."

~ Charles Swindoll

Stress is a natural part of being a human being and is a regular part of life.

What Happens When We Are Under Stress

When you are under stress your body creates a chain of chemical reactions that secrete "stress hormones" into the bloodstream, where they bring about specific physiological, psychological, and emotional changes that enhance the body's ability to deal with a threat—to either fight with or flee from it—which is the reason this response is often referred to as the emergency *fight-or-flight response*.

Your adrenal glands, located on your kidneys, release a surge of hormones, including adrenaline and cortisol. Adrenaline increases your heart rate, elevates your blood pressure, and boosts energy supplies. Cortisol, which can increase two- to five-fold during a stress response, gives you a quick burst of energy, heightens memory, and lowers your sensitivity to pain.

This is a perfect series of physiological responses if you are running through a thicket of bushes trying to get away from a bear. The combination of these things will allow you to make quick decisions like which way to go, help you get away quickly by giving you a burst of energy, and decrease any pain in the short term like being scratched by thorns or stepping on rocks. Or even the alternative—having to defend yourself and think and respond quickly to interactions with the threat.

The body is perfectly equipped for short fight-or-flight episodes that are quickly followed by periods of calm. The problem happens when your stress isn't triggered by a short event like being chased by an animal but rather long-term stressors like pending bills, a bad relationship, or an overbearing coworker or boss, and as a result you have too much cortisol being produced over a long period of time.

These daily and prolonged periods elevate levels of cortisol in the bloodstream and have been shown to have major negative health effects, such as blood sugar imbalances, higher blood pressure, suppressed thyroid function, decreased cognitive performance, lower immunity and inflammatory response in the body, and increased abdominal fat. The inability to control stress not only increases your risk of disease; it can both increase your waistline and prevent you from losing weight.

But it's not about the stress as much as it's about how we handle the stress.

So how do you control stress when you can't control other people's actions? Control your response and, more importantly, continued response to it. Getting upset because a coworker was snarky in the morning may be a natural reaction, but allowing it to stay with you all day and then taking your negative attitude home at night is not normal or healthy. Holding on to worry, anger, and resentment is unhealthy for both your mind and body.

Here are some ways to learn how to let go and stress less.

Get HIIT!

I told you that this was a complete program to better health and there is a method to the madness. Not only is HIIT training going to give you all the physical benefits of exercise but it also helps you better deal with stress—all stress. Exercise is a form of physical stress, meaning it takes your body out of homeostasis. It's "good stress" but stress all the same. But this is the type of stress that results in positive reactions in your body. HIIT training in particular gives you bursts of short, intense physiological stress followed by periods of active rest. When you place your body under the variant levels of low- and high-intensity stress, you are actually training your autonomic nervous system to better handle periods of extreme stress.

Your autonomic nervous system is a combination of the sympathetic nervous system—the system that excites us—and the parasympathetic nervous system—the system that calms us down. Intentionally creating this cycle of physical stress helps create a habitual pattern to allow you to better handle stress in all aspects of your life. One study showed people who engaged in HIIT training produced fewer stress hormones, and the hormones returned to base level quicker than for those who did not exercise. Don't skip the recommended HIIT training suggested in this program. It's multi-purpose and essential to making a lifestyle transformation.

Breath

Seriously, this sounds very simple but it's overlooked so often. There are thousands of years of Tibetan traditions of breathing, but short of running away to live with monks, you can start by simply breathing. Focusing on your breath for as few as five minutes can begin a practice of mindfulness that helps you bounce back from stress quicker.

Remember, the goal is not to avoid stress. That's impossible. The goal is to return to a state of homeostasis or balance as quickly as you can.

As a type-A, go-go personality, I have a hard time sitting still. I am that person who still gets up at 7 a.m. on vacation to find things to do. I don't binge-watch TV unless I am seriously ill and physically can't get out of bed. I try to fit something productive in every part of my day. During a strength training workout, my headphones are often playing a motivational talk, and my hikes are accompanied by an audiobook. Needless to say I find it hard to simply do nothing.

But this constant need for productivity and my inability to sit still don't serve me well in all aspects of my life. It makes me want to solve every problem, spend hours—sometimes days—lamenting on how to do something, even when it's not in my control, so I had to learn to slow down.

There's tons of research on how mindfulness not only reduces stress but also builds an inner strength so that future stressors have less impact on our happiness and physical well-being. How?

Neuroimaging research shows increased connectivity in the brain regions involved in attention, emotional control, emotional processing, and self-awareness—the prefrontal cortex—and decreased in the area of the brain associated with the threat response—the amygdala. One study by Dr. Richard Davidson, researcher and founder of the Center for Healthy Minds at the University of Wisconsin, Madison, showed that mindfulness helps us recover quicker between stressful events so that stress hormones don't build.

What Is Mindfulness?

Mindfulness is not sitting down for hours meditating. Rather, it's time you engage your brain in an intentional, nonjudgmental focus on the present moment. It can be as intense as silent, prolonged meditation or as simple as paying attention to your breath. One of the simplest exercises is "mindful breathing."

I began a practice of mindful breathing with only ten breaths, because that was all I could focus on. Every morning I would sit after morning prayer and simply spend a few minutes focusing my awareness on the physical sensations of my breath—pushing out the to-do list for the day or the bills that had to be paid or the meetings that had to be attended or the piles of clothes that had to be folded. Just my breath.

I find mindful breathing one of the simplest ways to introduce mindfulness to clients because it's not just simple—obviously everyone can do it—but it also includes physical sensations which you can connect to in a tangible way.

In the beginning you will not be successful. You will have to train your brain almost like you train a puppy. Sit. Sit. Sit. Your brain, like the puppy, will initially make several attempts to stray, but the gentle pull of refocusing will eventually become habit upon command.

Being the type-A person I am, I eventually figured out that forty-eight intentional breaths was five minutes of mindful breathing, and that became my daily goal. Some days, my puppy is constantly scampering off, but I gently remind her to sit over and over again. And some days she is still, focused, and present. Either way, I feel accomplished because I took the time for the process.

How to start a mindful breathing practice:

> Choose a time of day for your practice. In the beginning choose a time that you can be consistent, where you will be in the same place at the same time each day.

> Decide on a reasonable amount of time you can dedicate to begin your practice on a daily basis. Again, this does not have to be hours or even minutes. You can plan breaths if you want to. Give yourself a "low-hanging fruit" to begin with by starting with a small number. You can always increase it later or on the days you feel more focused.

> Choose a space. Find a space of quiet and comfort where you won't be disturbed. This can literally be anywhere—a corner of a room, the backyard, heck, if you're a mom of toddlers and your only quiet spot is the bathroom during nap time, use that. But create a dedicated space to your practice. If being in the same space is not possible, I recommend you get a mat or prayer rug and dedicate that to your mindfulness practice. When you sit on the mat, you are present. No matter where you are, the space within that may become your quiet space.

How to do mindful breathing:

> Sit or lie in a comfortable position. Pay attention to your body. Depress your shoulder blades, relax your spine, and allow your arms to drape to the side or place your hands in your lap and let them naturally fall open.

> Set a timer if you are doing it by time. Decide on the number of breaths if you are counting breaths.

> Breathe in through your nose and out through slightly pursed lips. Do not force the inhale or the exhale. Simply breathe.

Breathing cues:

> Pay attention to the feeling of the air coming into your nose when you inhale. Can you feel it in the back of your throat or does it warm to body temperature by then?

> Notice how the air flows from your mouth, how parched your lips are, if you are forcing it (don't) or if it flows naturally.

> How is your chest and your belly reacting to your lungs filling up, then deflating? Does it rise and fall slightly or dramatically?

> What is happening to your spine while you are breathing? Does your position change with the inhale or exhale?

> Notice the small intricacies of your moment related to where the breath is in the cycle.

Be Grateful

Stress is not just about events that happen to you or around you; it's also a mind-set that creates an emotional state that results in physiological response. The more stressed you are, the worse you feel about both your environment and yourself. Stress releases a multitude of toxic emotions, from envy and resentment to frustration and regret. Negativity and self-pity are ways that our views can sabotage our health and our happiness.

Gratitude, on the other hand, helps you feel more positive emotions, relish good experiences, improve your health, deal with adversity, and build strong relationships. Gratitude actually trains your brain to view life in a positive light. Research has shown that people who feel gratitude are happier, report more life satisfaction, and report less stress.

How often have you woken up "on the wrong side of the bed," when everything seems wrong with the world. You can no longer fit the pants you bought six months ago and you get dressed anyway. You make a cup of coffee just to knock it over and have to make a second. Then you go about your day, getting stuck in traffic, missing a project deadline, and being highly irritated at the comment your coworker made in the meeting you didn't want to be in. The end of the workday rolls around, and you are still feeling crappy about everything from your job to the state of political affairs. Those negative emotions can build up to create chronic stress that adversely affects your health and well-being.

The connection between gratitude and stress may not be immediately obvious, but here is how it works: In its simplest form gratitude distracts your attention from the negative to the positive. It's hard to think about two things at once, so being grateful allows your mind to focus on the good and pulls you out of your negative mind-set. By expressing gratitude, you give your thinking a more positive target.

When, for example, you express gratitude by recognizing that you have people in your life who care for you, it can enhance your sense of self-worth, increase self-esteem, and reduce levels of negative self-talk and thoughts.

Gratitude can mean different things to different people. In its simplest form, it can be saying thank you for a gift or service. For you it may mean feeling thankful when you have a near-miss or get over something bad that happened to you. But let's be clear, being grateful doesn't mean sticking your head in the sand and pretending like bad things don't happen; it simply means placing more attention on the good. It doesn't make you deny your feelings of stress or frustration. It simply means not allowing those feelings to linger and take over.

Gratitude simply asks that while we allow ourselves to feel what we feel, we *also* don't take for granted the many blessings that make our daily experience possible—that we notice the silver lining around the clouds. Instead of being irritated at spilling your coffee, take a minute to be thankful you actually have the ability to make a second cup. While you are frustrated at being stuck in a traffic jam, take a minute to imagine life without cars and how many benefits this convenience provides us. Instead of lamenting over how much you hate your job, think about all the skills you have that got you the position in the first place. There is always a silver lining; it's up to you to notice it.

Here are some ways to cultivate an attitude of gratitude.

Keep a gratitude journal. Keeping a gratitude journal is a great way to start reflecting on the positive things in your life. It doesn't have to be an entire notebook dedicated to paragraphs of things you are grateful for. Simply make it a habit to write a few sentences of gratitude at the end of each day and silently acknowledge all that you have. It can be a part of your fitness journal or even in the note section of your daily calendar. Researchers Emmons and McCullough (2003) found participants who kept gratitude journals reported higher levels of optimism, felt better about their lives as a whole, were more likely to have made progress toward important personal goals, exercised more regularly, and reported fewer negative health symptoms.

Write a thank-you note. Having meaningful relationships in our life leads to a deeper sense of contentment and happiness. You can make yourself happier and nurture your relationship with another person by writing a thank-you letter expressing your enjoyment and appreciation of that person's impact on your life. Studies show that when you thank people for their presence and contribution to your life, it fosters lasting relationships. Send a thank-you email, write a note, or better yet, deliver and read it in person if possible. Make a habit of sending at least one gratitude note a month. At least twice a year write one to yourself.

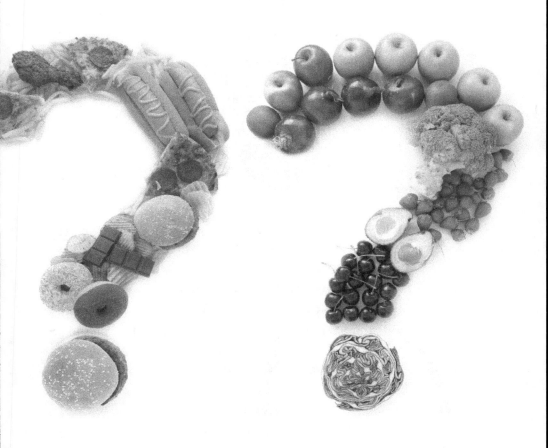

Chapter 11:

But Wait...
I Have Some Questions

Keto FAQ

Is the keto diet just another name for the Atkins diet?

Don't be confused, they are not the same. The Atkins diet is low in carbohydrates and high in protein, while the keto diet is low in carbohydrates, high in fat, and moderate in protein. Lowering carb intakes alone cannot activate nutritional ketosis. You can only truly change the body energy source from glucose to fat by increasing fat consumption.

I thought eating fat was bad! Won't eating fat raise my cholesterol?

Good question! This is a common mistaken belief. Properly formatted low-carb ketogenic diets have been proven to lower LDL, which is the "bad" cholesterol and increase HDL, which is the "good" cholesterol,

I LOVE bread and have serious sugar cravings! Can keto help?

Yes. Bread converts into sugar in the body so bread addiction is sugar addiction. When you eat according to the mR40 method, you will enjoy delicious, nutrient-dense foods with lots of healthy fats which helps you feel satisfied and eliminates the incessant craving for sweets.

Why can't I eat berries and oranges in phase I of the program?

Although both foods are allowed in Phase II of the program due to their anti-angiogenesis properties, Phase I of your program should consist of foods that are both angiogenesis inhibiting AND low on the glycemic load. Because berries are easily overconsumed which can add extra sugar to your diet, I recommend that you eliminate them in phase I of the program to stay below twenty grams of carbs a day.

Will I ever be able to eat fruit again?

Yes. In phase II of the mR40 method, you are encouraged to incorporate angiogenesis inhibiting , low-glycemic load fruits into your diet. In addition after your initial forty days, it's recommended that you allow yourself a "flex day" a couple of times a month in which you can eat anything you like.

Is this just another fad diet?

Not at all. The ketogenic diet has been around for a hundred years, and many people have been using it for its many health benefits. Besides its use to reduce body weight, the keto diet is also used to manage complications from diabetes, Parkinson's disease, Alzheimer's disease, PCOS, metabolic syndrome, and many more. Intermittent fasting has been used literally for thousands of years for both its physical and spiritual benefits. The reason keto is so widely used is because it is more than a diet; it is a lifestyle that inspires a total positive change in people.

Is this another complicated meal plan that's hard to follow?

There are many keto plans that are complicated. They are poor plans that do not explain the procedures clearly, so the users do not have positive results because they fail to attain ketosis. This system is different. We took the time to create several varieties of easy-to-make meals, including pescatarian and vegetarian options.

I presently have a health condition. Is it safe to try out keto?

I would advise you to consult your health-care professional before incorporating this or any other dietary and exercises changes. It's highly recommend that you consult your doctor if you are breastfeeding, have type 1 diabetes or a kidney-related disease.

AI Foods FAQ

Will AI foods prevent me from getting cancer?

Currently the answer to that question is no, but research is still ongoing. What we do know is that it's a good idea to use angiogenesis-inhibiting foods as a component of a healthy diet while being treated for cancer.

Should I eat AI foods every day?

Yes. The current research is showing that having angiogenesis-inhibiting compounds on a regular basis is where the benefit happens.

Will I lose weight if I eat AI foods but don't eat keto?

That depends on a lot of factors not covered in this book. No matter what plan you choose to follow, AI foods listed in this book are beneficial foods to incorporate into your diet.

Intermittent Fasting FAQ

Isn't intermittent fasting just another way of starving myself?

No. Intermittent fasting is not about reducing calories. You eat the same amount you would during a normal day except you only eat during a certain window of time. It's a version of nutrient timing that changes the way your body metabolizes food. Combined with high amounts of healthy fats, you won't feel hungry and will force your body to burn fat as fuel.

mR40 method FAQ

I have tried just about every other type of diet. Will this really work?

Yes. I have seen many people (especially women) yo-yo between diets and eating plans that don't work for them and they are at the verge of losing hope. But when they gave my program a try, they began to see amazing results and fall in love with my mR40 method of keto. This method has worked for me and hundreds of other people all over the world.

I am a vegetarian. Can I use your program?

Of course, you can. The animal protein options can be easily replaced with your favorite plant-based proteins. In addition I have included many vegetarian options.

I am allergic to gluten. Will this program work for me?

This program is perfect for you. Because keto diets cut down on carb intakes, by eliminating grains the meals are totally gluten-free.

What if I don't like some of the meals in the diet plan?

There are many healthy keto-friendly meal options in the mR40 method meal plan. You can simply choose any one of them to replace the ones you do not like.

Can I drink coffee?

Yes. If you feel like you cannot get through your day without multiple cups of coffee, I would recommend that you use a couple days over the weekend (or when you are off work/ school) to detox off coffee and break your addiction. However, if you only drink one cup a day, that's perfectly acceptable. BUT... there is a but. You must drink it black during your detox process, no milk (not even milk substitutes) and no sweetener or sugar alternatives.

What if I am allergic to or don't like an ingredient?

Don't eat it. One of the things I emphasize in this program is to listen to your body.

What if I am still hungry?

If you are still hungry, then eat until you are satisfied. There are no set portions. Review the chapter in this book on mindful eating to guide your intake.

What if I'm not hungry?

Eat a snack-size portion or don't eat at all. But remember not to wait until you are starving. Part of this journey is listening to your body.

Should I continue my medication during the detox?

Yes. Never stop doctor-prescribed medication without consulting your medical provider.

Should I take supplements?

It's up to you. I support everyone taking a good whole-food multivitamin every day. I also believe we can effectively detox without lots of supplements, teas, and gimmicks. However, if you feel your supplements are an important part of your healthy lifestyle, then continue to take them.

I can't start right away! I am afraid I will fail to complete the plan.

Although you have the responsibility to follow the plan, I designed this program with the beginner in mind. The method contains several tips that can help you get back on track quickly when you fall off or stop progressing.

We are all imperfect humans and will slip off every so often. With my tips, you can get back to your healthy lifestyle as quickly as possible.

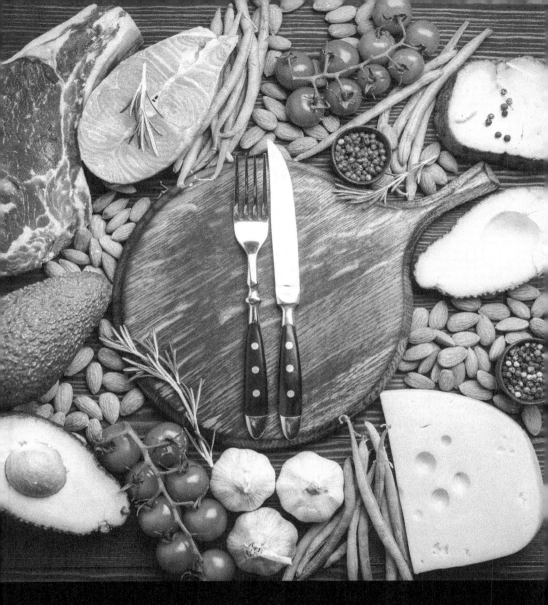

Chapter 12:

Seven-Day Meal Plan

ollowing a low-carb eating plan isn't really difficult nor is it limiting. Just eat whole foods. When you begin, eat as simply as possible. Don't attempt to make fancy cookie and cake substitutes or buy pre-made keto products. Keto food is whole food. There will be a time when you can try your hand at keto cinnamon rolls (yes, that's a thing), but for the first forty days at least, keep your foods and meal planning simple.

There are simple substitutions for foods you may have been used to eating, like using cauliflower for rice (cauliflower can substitute for LOTS of cooked grain- and potato-based dishes by the way, so make it a staple on your grocery list). But just as people who follow a vegan lifestyle get used to substitutions like seitan for actual meat, you, too, will get used to things like cauliflower mashed potatoes.

Below is just an example of what a one-week, low-carb mR40 plan can look like. These meals are not set in stone and you don't have to eat these exact meals. They are some of my favorite meals, because of both taste and simplicity.

You'll notice with the meal plan below there are two meals and one optional snack each day. Since you will be following a schedule of intermittent fasting during the forty-day mR40 plan, there is no need to try to squeeze three meals into your day. Eat when you are hungry and stop when you are satisfied. Pay attention to your body and be cognizant of your environment and social cues. Don't eat just because you have access to food, or because you feel like it's "time" for you to eat. For this same reason I rarely include portion sizes in the meal plan. It's important that you choose foods that nourish your body, and eat with purpose.

Your First Seven Days on the mR40 Method.

Day 1 - Sunday

5:00 PM - Stop Eating

Day 2 - Monday

Fast: 24 hours

Exercise: Morning Fasted Cardio – 90-Minute Walk

During the Day: Water, Black Coffee, Black Tea, or Herbal Tea With No Sugar

5:00 PM - Keto Coffee / Chai

Meal 1 - Seared Salmon with Sautéed Spinach

8:00 PM - Stop Eating

Day 3 - Tuesday

Fast: 20 hours

Exercise: Morning Fasted Cardio – 60-Minute Walk

During the Day: Water, Black Coffee, Black Tea, or Herbal Tea With No Sweetener

5:00 PM

Keto Coffee / Chai

Meal 1: Bok Choy and Turkey Stir-fry, Cauliflower Mashed Potatoes

Snack (Optional - See snack list)

8:00 PM - Stop Eating

Day 4 - Wednesday

Fast: 16 hours

Exercise: Whatever time works in your schedule - HIIT Routine

During the Day: Water, Black Coffee, Black Tea or Herbal Tea With No Sweetener

12:00 PM - Break Fast

Meal 1:

Keto Coffee / Chai

Scrambled Eggs and Keto Hash Brown

Snack (Optional - See snack list)

Meal 2: Vegetarian Keto Lasagna and Salad

8:00 PM - Stop Eating

Day 5 - Thursday

Fast: 16 hours

Exercise: Morning Fasted Cardio - 30-60 minutes

During the Day: Water, Black Coffee, Black Tea or Herbal Tea With No Sweetener

12:00 PM - Break Fast

Meal 1:

Keto Coffee / Chai

Loaded Veggie Omelet

Snack (Optional - See snack list)

Meal 2: Crispy Curry Rubbed Chicken and Yellow "Rice"

8:00 PM - Stop Eating

Day 6 - Friday

Fast: 16 hours

Exercise: Whatever time works in your schedule - HIIT Routine

During the Day: Water, Black Coffee, Black Tea or Herbal Tea With No Sweetener

12:00 PM - Break Fast

Meal 1:

Keto Coffee / Chai

2 Turkey Patties and ½ Chopped Avocado

Snack (Optional - See snack list)

Meal 2: Garlic Butter Steelhead Trout and Mashed Cauliflower "Potatoes"

8:00 PM - Stop Eating

Day 7 - Saturday

Fast: 16 hours

Exercise: No Exercise / Rest Day

During the Day: Water, Black Coffee, Black Tea or Herbal Tea With No Sweetener

12:00 PM - Break Fast

Meal 1:

Keto Coffee / Chai

2 Scrambled eggs with Cheese between 2 Keto Flatbread

Snack (Optional - See snack list)

Meal 2: Keto Fried Chicken and Cauliflower "Mac N Cheese"

8:00 PM - Stop Eating

Day 8 - Sunday

Fast: 16 hours

Exercise: 60 minutes Active Rest / Do something you enjoy that includes movement. Hike, play soccer with your kids, go for stroll on the beach.

During the Day: Water, Black Coffee, Black Tea or Herbal Tea With No Sweetener

12:00 PM - Break Fast

Meal 1:

Keto Coffee / Chai

Spinach Mozzarella Stuffed Burgers

Snack (Optional - See snack list)

Meal 2:

Caveman Chili and Keto "Cornbread"

8:00 PM - Stop Eating

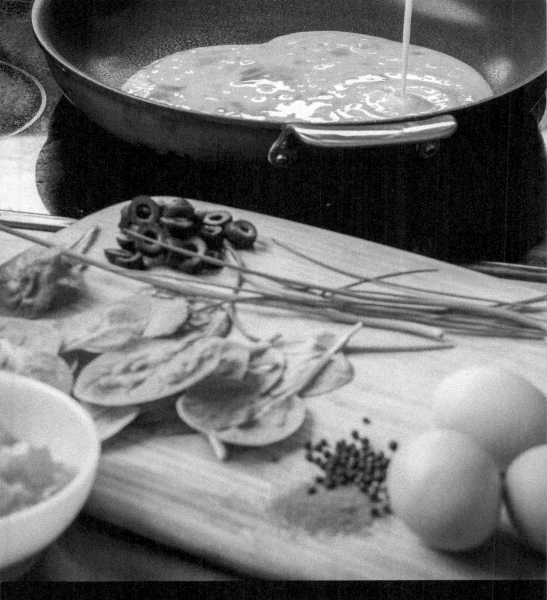

Chapter 13:

Food and Recipes

Hot Beverages

mR40 Keto Coffee

Ingredients

    1 package of Starbucks Instant Coffee (or 1 cup prepared coffee)

    1 tbsp. unsalted butter (hormone free)

    1 tbsp. coconut oil

    1 tbsp. collagen

Directions

Place instant coffee granules, butter, coconut oil, and collagen in high-powered blender (NutriBullet or similar)

Add 1 cup hot water. Blend until well combined and you see froth forming.

Per Serving: 273 Calories, 30g Fats, 1g Net Carbs, and 0g Protein

mR40 Keto Chai

Ingredients

    1 cup prepared chai tea (from teabag)

    1 tbsp. unsalted butter (hormone free)

    1 tbsp. coconut oil

    1 tbsp. collagen

Directions

Place chai tea, butter, coconut oil, and collagen in high-powered blender (NutriBullet or similar).

Blend until well combined and you see froth forming.

Breakfast Options

Loaded Veggie Omelet

Ingredients

 1 tsp. olive oil or avocado oil

 2 tbsp. chopped red bell pepper

 1 tbsp. chopped onion

 ¼ cup sliced mushrooms

 ½ cup loosely packed fresh baby spinach leaves, rinsed

 ½ cup baby kale leaves rinsed and chopped

 ½ cup 2 eggs, beaten

 1 tbsp. water

 Dash salt

 Dash pepper

 1 tbsp. shredded cheddar cheese

Directions

In 8-inch nonstick skillet, heat oil over medium-high heat. Add bell pepper, onion, and mushrooms to oil. Cook 2 minutes, stirring frequently, until onion is tender. Stir in spinach and kale; continue cooking and stirring just until greens wilt. Remove vegetables from pan to small bowl.

In medium bowl, beat egg product, water, salt and pepper with fork or whisk until well mixed. Reheat same skillet over medium-high heat. Quickly pour egg mixture into pan. While sliding pan back and forth rapidly over heat, quickly stir with spatula to spread eggs continuously over bottom of pan as they thicken. Let stand over heat a few seconds to lightly brown bottom of omelet. Do not overcook; omelet will continue to cook after folding.

Place cooked vegetable mixture over half of omelet; top with cheese. With spatula, fold other half of omelet over vegetables. Gently slide out of pan onto plate. Serve immediately.

Keto Hash Brown

Ingredients

1 head cauliflower (shredded/riced using a food processor or grater)

½ large onion (shredded using a food processor or grater)

2 tbsp. golden flaxseed meal

½ tsp. garlic salt (or sea salt)

1 large egg

½ large egg white (see instructions)

Oil for frying

Directions

Steam riced cauliflower for 3-5 minutes, until tender. (Alternatively, microwave it for 1-3 minutes until tender.) Set aside to cool.

While cauliflower is cooling, whisk together the shredded onion, golden flaxseed meal, garlic salt, egg, and one egg white in a large bowl.

When the riced cauliflower is cool enough to handle, wrap it in a cheesecloth or towel. Squeeze tightly over the sink to drain as much moisture as possible. Stir the cauliflower into the bowl with the other ingredients.

Tip: If it doesn't stick together well when trying to form a patty, add another egg white to help it stick.

Heat a generously oiled skillet over medium heat. Drop heaping tablespoonfuls of the cauliflower mixture onto the pan and press down with a spatula to form hash brown patties. Cook for 2-4 minutes, until the bottom is browned, then flip and repeat for 2-4 minutes on the other side. Repeat with the remaining cauliflower mixture.

Depending on the size of the scoops, this can make between 12 and 18 hash brown patties.

Serving Suggestion: Serve with 2 scrambled eggs

Breakfast Turkey Patties

Makes 4 servings

<u>Ingredients</u>

    2 lbs. ground turkey

    1/4 cup minced onion

    1/4 cup minced red pepper

<u>Seasoning</u>

    1 1/2 tsp. rubbed sage

    ½ tsp. thyme

    ½ tsp black seed (optional)

    1 tsp. ground pepper

    1 1/2 tsp. sea salt

    1 1/2 tsp. parsley flakes

    ¼ tsp. red pepper flakes

    ¼ tsp. ground nutmeg

<u>Directions</u>

Cook onions and pepper until onions are translucent. Set aside to cool.

Combine spices together. In large bowl combine completely cooled onion mix, spice mix, and 2 pounds of ground turkey. Mix well. (You can cook it right away, but it tastes better if you refrigerate it for 3 to 24 hours to let the flavors blend together.)

Shape into 2-inch patties and cook in pan 3 minutes on each side OR in a 350-degree oven, turning over after 3 minutes.

Lunch / Dinner

Spinach Mozzarella Stuffed Burgers

Makes 4 patties, enough for 4 people

Ingredients

    1½ lbs. ground chuck

    1 tsp. salt

    ¾ tsp. ground black pepper

    2 cups fresh spinach, firmly packed

    ½ cup shredded mozzarella cheese (about 4 oz)

    2 tbsp. grated Parmesan cheese

Directions

In a medium bowl, combine ground beef, salt, and pepper. Scoop about ¼ cup of mixture and with dampened hands shape into 8 patties about ½-inch thick. Place in the refrigerator.

Place spinach in saucepan over medium-high heat. Cover and cook for 2 minutes, until wilted.

Drain and let cool. With your hands squeeze the spinach to extract as much liquid as possible.

Transfer to a cutting board, chop the spinach, and place in a bowl. Stir in mozzarella cheese and Parmesan. Scoop about ¼ cup of stuffing and mound in the center of 4 patties. Cover with remaining 4 patties, and seal the edges by pressing firmly together. Cup each patty with your hands to round out the edges, and press on the top to flatten slightly into a single thick patty.

Heat a grill or a grill pan to medium high (if you're using an outdoor grill, lightly oil the grill grates). Grill burgers for 5 to 6 minutes on each side.

Serving Suggestion: Eat alone as an open-faced burger or place between a split keto bun (page_____) topped with lettuce, tomato, and ½ sliced cucumber.

Keto Fried Chicken

Ingredients:

    1 whole chicken, cut up

    2 large eggs, beaten

    1 tbsp. kosher salt

    1 tsp. black pepper

    1 tsp. paprika

    ½ tsp. dried mustard powder

    ½ tsp. garlic powder

    ½ tsp. onion powder

    Coating Flour

    1 cup coconut flour

    2 cups almond flour

    1 tsp. kosher salt

    ½ tsp. black pepper

    ½ tsp. paprika

    ¼ tsp. dried mustard powder

    ¼ tsp. garlic powder

    ¼ tsp. onion powder

    Peanut oil, for frying

Directions

Combine the chicken and eggs in a bowl. Turn the chicken to coat with eggs. Add in all the seasonings. Mix well to ensure all the chicken is coated with the seasonings. Place flour and coating seasoning inside a Ziploc bag. Place chicken pieces a few at a time in the bag and shake until coated.

Heat the oil to 360 degrees. Shake off all of the excess flour. Then, add in the chicken and fry on both sides until golden brown. Place cooked chicken in a strainer lined with paper towels to drain off excess oil. Serve while the chicken is still warm.

Bok Choy Stir Fry with Ground Turkey

Ingredients:

    2 tsp. cooking oil

    1/2 pound ground turkey

    1 stalk green onion, chopped

    2 tsp. grated fresh ginger

    2 cloves garlic, finely minced

    1 pound bok choy, stems chopped and separated from chopped greens

    1 tbsp. water

    2 tsp. soy sauce

    1 tsp. sesame oil

Directions:

In a wok or large sauté pan over high heat, add the cooking oil. When hot, add ground turkey and sauté until browned (but not fully cooked through). Lower heat to medium high and add green onion, ginger, and garlic and stir for 30 seconds or until fragrant.

Add chopped bok choy stems and toss well to coat with the oil, aromatics, and turkey. Cover the wok. Allow to cook for 2 minutes or until the bok choy is crisp-tender. Add water and chopped bok choy greens and cook for 1 minute until they are bright green but slightly wilted.

Add soy sauce, sesame oil, and toss well for 30 seconds. The baby bok choy should be just tender in the stem, but not too soft. Serve immediately.

Serving Suggestion: Serve over a bed of cauliflower mashed potatoes.

Crispy Curry Rubbed Chicken Thigh

Makes 4 servings

<u>Ingredients</u>

> 4 chicken thighs
>
> 4 Tbsp. olive oil
>
> 2 tsp. yellow curry
>
> 2 tsp. salt
>
> 1 tsp. cumin
>
> 1 tsp. paprika
>
> 1 tsp. garlic powder
>
> 1/2 tsp. cayenne pepper
>
> 1/2 tsp. allspice
>
> 1/2 tsp. chili powder
>
> 1/2 tsp. coriander
>
> 1/8 cardamom
>
> 1/8 cinnamon
>
> 1/8 pinch ginger

<u>Directions</u>

Preheat oven to 425 F.

Mix together all spices into a bowl. Wrap a baking sheet in foil and lay chicken thighs on the foil.

Rub olive oil evenly into all chicken thighs. Rub spice mixture on both sides of the chicken, coating liberally.

Bake for 40-50 minutes. Let cool for 5 minutes before serving.

Serving Suggestion: Serve with keto yellow "rice"

Seared Salmon with Sautéed Spinach and Mushrooms

Servings: 8 servings (1.5 cups)

Ingredients

- 1 tbsp. olive oil
- 2 cloves garlic
- 1/2 lb. mushrooms
- 2 tbsp. butter
- 2 tomatoes
- 2 cups spinach
- salt and pepper
- 1 tbsp. balsamic vinegar
- 1 tbsp. olive oil
- 2 salmon fillets

Directions

Get your salmon fillets ready by patting them with a paper towel to get rid of any excess moisture. Season both sides with salt and pepper and keep them in the fridge while you prep the rest of the recipe.

Start by heating some olive oil over a medium heat and slicing the garlic, mushrooms, and tomatoes. We left ours pretty chunky. Cook the garlic and mushrooms in the olive oil until they've shrunken in size a bit. Add butter to the pan to get them nice and crispy. Then add the tomatoes and wait until they've denatured a bit. Add the spinach last and cook just until it has all wilted. Season with salt and pepper and toss well. Remove the veggies from the heat and onto a plate. Cover with foil while you cook the salmon.

Heat another tbsp. of olive oil in that same pan and wait until it's very, very hot. Lay the salmon fillets skin side down onto the pan and leave them to sear for about 4-5 minutes. Don't move them around or disturb them because you may end up breaking the fillets and you won't get that nice, even sear. Then flip the fillets and let them cook for another 4-5 minutes.

Lastly, uncover the veggies and drizzle them with some balsamic vinegar. Place the salmon fillets right on top and garnish with fresh lemon. Enjoy!

Ground Turkey, Ginger, and Garlic Bok Choy Stir-Fry

Servings: 8 servings (1.5 cups)

Ingredients

- 1 lb. ground turkey
- 5 bok choy stems from bunch
- 2 cloves of garlic, minced
- 1 tsp. fresh ginger, grated
- 2 tbsp. coconut oil
- salt to taste

Directions

Add 1 tbsp. of coconut oil into a saucepan (or wok) on medium heat, then add ground turkey. Stir frequently until turkey turns brown. Remove from pan and set aside in bowl

Cut off the ends of the bok choy and chop the bok choy into 1-inch-long chunks.

Add 1 tbsp. of coconut oil into the same saucepan (or wok) on medium heat, and then add the bok choy chunks. Stir frequently while the bok choy cooks.

After the bok choy starts to wilt, mix in the cooked ground turkey, garlic, ginger, and salt to taste.

Cook for another 1-2 minutes and serve.

Caveman Chili

Ingredients

2 lbs. marbled ground beef or ground turkey

1 medium onion

1 medium green pepper

1 cup beef broth

1/3 cup tomato paste

2 tbsp. soy sauce

2 tbsp. olive oil

8-10 tbsp. chili powder

1 1/2 tsp. cumin

2 tsp. minced garlic

2 tsp. paprika

1 tsp. oregano

1 tsp. cayenne pepper

1 tsp. Worcestershire

1 tsp. black pepper

1 tsp. salt

Directions

Chop pepper and onion into small pieces.

Combine all spices together to make sauce.

Sauté ground beef in a pan until browned, transfer to a slow cooker.

Sauté vegetables in olive oil until onions are translucent.

Add everything to the slow cooker and mix together.

Simmer for 2 1/2 hours on high, then simmer for 20-30 minutes without the top.

Serving Suggestion: Place chili in serving bowl and top with shredded cheddar cheese right before serving. Serve with keto cornbread (Page:)

Garlic Butter Steelhead Trout

Makes 4 servings

Ingredients

    1 pound steelhead trout filet, skin removed

    2 tbsp. butter

    1/2 lemon, juice squeezed

    1-2 cloves garlic, minced

    1 tsp. parsley, minced (optional)

    salt and pepper to taste

Directions

Preheat oven to 375° F.

Spray a sheet of aluminum foil with cooking spray and place the trout filet in the center. Fold up all 4 sides of the foil. Season trout with salt and pepper and then squeeze juice from half a lemon over the fish until covered.

Melt butter in microwave-safe bowl, stir in fresh minced garlic, and drizzle over the trout until evenly coated. Top with fresh minced parsley.

Fold the sides of the foil over the trout, covering completely, and seal into a closed packet. Place directly on oven rack and bake until cooked through, about 15-20 minutes.

Optional step: Open the foil exposing the top of the trout and broil for the last 4-5 minutes, for a browned top.

Vegetarian Keto Lasagna

Makes 6 servings

Ingredients

  2 medium eggplants (about 1 ½ lb.)

  1 cup marinara sauce

  fresh spinach (10.6 oz.) or frozen spinach (11.6 oz.)

  1 1/3 cup feta cheese

  1 cup mozzarella cheese, grated

  ½ cup Parmesan cheese, grated

  6 large eggs

  ¼ cup + 2 tbsp. ghee

  ½ tsp. salt or more to taste

Directions

Preheat the oven to 200 C / 400 F. Slice the eggplant into 1/2 inch (~ 1 cm) slices and place on a baking tray. Grease with 1/4 of melted ghee, season with a pinch of salt, and place in the oven. Cook for about 20 minutes.

If you're using frozen spinach, let it defrost at room temperature for a couple of hours (or microwave). If you're using fresh spinach, you'll need to blanch it. Bring a pot of water to a boil over high heat. Fill a bowl with ice and water or simply with cold water. Place the spinach leaves into the boiling water and cook for 30-60 seconds. Transfer the leaves immediately into the iced water using tongs or a strainer. Once they cool down, remove the leaves from the cold water. Drain the excess water by placing the spinach in a strainer and squeezing the excess fluids out.

Meanwhile, prepare the marinara sauce.

When the eggplant is done, remove from the oven and set aside. Reduce the temperature to 180 C / 360 F. Prepare the omelets. Crack one egg at a time in a bowl, season with a pinch of salt, and mix well.

Pour in a hot pan greased with ghee (use the remaining 2 tbsp. of ghee for greasing the pan as needed) and swirl around to create a very thin omelet. Cook for just about a minute or two, until the top is firm. Place on a plate and repeat for the remaining eggs. Make a total of 6 omelets. Start assembling the lasagna by placing a layer of 2 omelets on the bottom of a 9 x12 baking dish.

TIP: You can create fewer layers if you like—it's totally up to you. Just make sure you top the lasagna with some mozzarella and Parmesan.

Spread a third of the marinara sauce on top of the omelets. Add a third of the eggplant slices, a third of the grated mozzarella cheese, half of the spinach, and half of the crumbled feta cheese. Top with 2 more omelets.

Repeat layering the lasagna: Spread a third of the marinara sauce on top, add a third of the eggplant slices, and a third of grated mozzarella. Add the remaining spinach and feta cheese. For the last layer, add the remaining omelets, marinara sauce, eggplant slices and mozzarella cheese. Top with all of the grated Parmesan cheese and place in the oven. Bake for 25-30 minutes. When done, the top should be crispy and golden brown. Remove from the oven and set aside to cool down. Cut into 6 pieces / servings.

NOTE: Eat immediately or let it cool down and store in the fridge for up to 5 days. The lasagna can be served either warm or cold.

Serve with salad and olive oil-based dressing.

Sides

Cauliflower Mashed "Potatoes"

Ingredients

1 head cauliflower

3 tbsp. milk

1 tbsp. butter

2 tbsp. light sour cream

1/4 tsp. garlic salt

freshly ground black pepper

snipped chives

Directions

Separate the cauliflower into florets and discard the core.

Bring about 2 cups of water to a simmer in a pot, then add the cauliflower. Cover and turn the heat to medium. Cook the cauliflower for 12-15 minutes or until very tender.

Drain and discard all of the water (the drier the cauliflower, the better) and add the milk, butter, sour cream, salt and pepper, and mash with a masher until it looks like mashed potatoes. Top with chives.

Yellow "Rice"

<u>Ingredients</u>

 2 cups riced cauliflower

 2 tbsp. butter

 ½ tsp. salt

 ½ tsp. dried parsley

 ½ tsp. ground cumin

 1 tsp. turmeric

 2 garlic cloves, sliced

Preheat the oven to 350°F (175°C).

Using a grater or grater attachment on a food processor, shred the cauliflower.

Combine all of the ingredients on a sheet pan and toss together until all of the riced cauliflower is yellow.

Spread the seasoned rice out evenly over the sheet pan.

Roast on the bottom rack for 20 minutes.

Remove from the oven. Use a thin spatula to scrape it up and mix it all together.

Cauliflower Mac n Cheese

Servings: 8 servings (3/4 cup)

Ingredients

    2 pounds frozen cauliflower florets

    1 cup heavy whipping cream

    4 ounces cream cheese, cubed

    8 ounces cheddar cheese, shredded

    1 tsp. Dijon mustard

    1 tsp. turmeric

    ½ tsp. powdered garlic

    Salt and pepper to taste

Directions

Cook the cauliflower florets according to the package instructions.

Bring the cream to a simmer. Use a whisk to stir in the cream cheese and mix until smooth.

Stir in 6 ounces of the shredded cheddar cheese. Save the other 2 ounces for later. Mix until the cheese melts into the sauce. Add the Dijon mustard, turmeric, powdered garlic, salt, and pepper. The sauce will become a smooth yellow color.

Make sure that the cauliflower is drained, then add it to the cheese sauce. Evenly coat the florets with sauce. Sprinkle on the remaining 2 ounces of cheddar cheese, then stir until mostly melted.

"Breads"

Keto Buns

Makes 12 servings

<u>Dry Ingredients:</u>

    1 ½ cup almond flour (150 g/ 5.3 oz.)

    1/3 cup psyllium husk powder (40 g/ 1.4 oz.)

    ½ cup coconut flour (60 g/ 2.1 oz.)

    ½ cup flax meal (75 g/ 2.6 oz.)

    1 tsp. garlic powder

    1 tsp. onion powder

    2 tsp. cream of tartar

    1 tsp. baking soda

    1 tsp. salt

    5 tbsp. sesame or 1-2 tbsp caraway seeds

<u>Wet Ingredients:</u>

    6 large egg whites

    2 large eggs

    2 cups boiling water

<u>Directions</u>

Preheat the oven to 350 F / 175 C.

Use scales to measure all the ingredients carefully.

Do not use whole psyllium husks. If you cannot find psyllium husk powder, use a blender or coffee grinder and process until fine.

Mix all the dry ingredients apart from the sesame seeds in a bowl (almond flour, coconut flour, ground flaxseed, psyllium powder, garlic and onion powder, baking soda, cream of tartar and salt). Add wet ingredients and blend well until wet and fluffy. Scoop with ice cream scoop onto a cookie sheet 3 inches apart.

Press down slightly for flatter buns.

Bake for 45-50 minutes. Cool and serve.

These are great all-purpose buns. They can be used as hamburger buns, breakfast buns served with cream cheese or butter, or any meal side.

Notes:

You can use 2 teaspoons of gluten-free baking powder instead of baking soda and cream of tartar.

Make sure you use a kitchen scale for measuring all the dry ingredients. Using just cups may not be enough to achieve best results, especially in baked goods. Weights per cups and tablespoons may vary depending on the product/brand or if you make your own ingredients (like flax meal from flax seeds). Psyllium absorbs lots of water. When baking with psyllium, you must remember to drink enough water throughout the day to prevent constipation!

Keto Flat Bread (Naan)

Ingredients:

½ cup almond flour

2 tbsp. psyllium husk

2 tsp. baking powder.

½ cup hot water

Directions

Mix dry ingredients. Add water. Combine with your hands to make small balls. Pat flat with your hands OR roll between parchment paper and use a pot top to cut round shapes. Cook in an oiled pan for 3 minutes on each side

Keto Cornbread

Ingredients

2 cups almond flour

¼ cup coconut flour

3 tsp baking powder

1 tsp kosher salt

3 large eggs

½ cup butter, melted

¼ cup sour cream

1/3 cup monk fruit sweetener

Directions

Preheat the oven to 350 degrees.

In a large bowl, combine the flours, baking powder, and salt. Mix in the eggs, butter, sour cream, and monk fruit sweetener. (I prefer monk fruit for baking, as it blends and tastes better in the finished product.) The batter may appear think but it will bake wonderfully.

Butter and dust a cast-iron skillet with almond flour. Put the batter in the skillet and bake for 20-25 minutes or until golden brown. Spread butter on the top of the hot cornbread immediately after it comes out of the oven and let it cool slightly before cutting.

Keto Snack Ideas

- **Avocados:** GREAT choice because they're a whole food and very easy to eat "as is." Just add a little salt and pepper and you're golden.

- Beef and turkey bacon: Cook some ahead of time to have on hand for snacks on the go.

- Beef jerky: Make sure the brand you choose is no- or very low-carb with few added ingredients. Be wary of anything with added sugars, as that will kick up the carb content.

- Cherry tomatoes

- Cocoa nibs: These are a nice low-carb alternative to chocolate chips!

- Fat bombs (a combination of ingredients such as butter, coconut oil, nuts and seeds that can be used as a snack meal replacement or side dish): Stuffed with healthy fats and so easy to make at home! Store in the freezer right after making, then keep in a travel cooler until ready to eat.

- Iced coffee: Drink it black (no added sugars) or only with full-fat milk or cream or MCT oil powder.

- Kale chips: If buying these, look for no added sugars—or make them yourself at home using coconut oil or ghee.

- Nuts, nut butters, or seeds: Remember, some nuts are fairly high in carbs (like peanuts, cashews, and pistachios). Choose higher fat choices, such as almonds or macadamia nuts, and seeds high in omega 3s like flaxseed and chia.

- Pepperoni slices: These are highly processed, so limit them and try to find organic and hormone-free if possible. Great paired with a high-fat cheese.

- Sardines: Not only do these provide a healthy dose of fat and other nutrients, they're also zero carb. Sardines are highly recommended by keto gurus Dom D'Agostino and Tim Ferriss.

- Seaweed snacks: Make sure there aren't any added ingredients that contribute extra carbs.

- Stevia-sweetened dark chocolate: If not sweetened with stevia, make sure it's at least 80 percent cocoa content or higher, as the carbs can add up quickly otherwise.

- String cheese: Make sure it's the full-fat version without added carbs or other fillers.

- Olives

- Veggie sticks: Slice your favorite keto-friendly veggies and store in the fridge so they're easy to grab and go. You could dip these in homemade guacamole or eat with full-fat cheeses.

Comprehensive mR40 Food List

Proteins

Albacore tuna
Anchovies
Bass
Beef
Bone Marrow
Chicken
Chicken Livers
Cod
Eel
Eggs
Goat
Haddock
Halibut
Hearts
Herring
Kidney
Lake Trout
Lamb
Liver
Mackerel
Mahi Mahi
Ox Liver
Perch
Red Snapper
Rockfish
Salmon
Sardines
Shellfish
Swordfish
Tongue

Tuna
Turkey

Vegetables

Artichoke Hearts
Arugula
Asparagus
Avocado
Bamboo Shoots
Beet Greens
Bell Peppers
Bok Choy
Broccoli
Broccoli Rabe
Brussels Sprouts
Cabbage
Cauliflower
Celery
Chard
Collards
Cucumbers
Daikon
Dandelion greens
Eggplant
Endive
Fennel Root
Garlic
Green Beans
Iceberg Lettuce
Kale
Kimchi
Kohlrabi

Leeks
Mixed Vegetables
Mushrooms
Mung Bean Sprouts
Mustard Greens
Napa Cabbage
Nori
Olives
Onions
Peas
Peppers (all kinds)
Purslane
Radish
Red Cabbage
Romaine Lettuce
Sauerkraut
Seaweed (nori)
Spinach
Summer Squash
Swiss Chard
Tomatoes
Turnip Greens
Watercress
Yellow Pepper
Zucchini
Acorn Squash*
Beets*
Butternut Squash*
Carrots*
Jicama*
Parsnips*

Pumpkin*
Squash*
Sweet Potato*
Yam*

Fats/Oils
Avocado
Butter (Grass Fed)
Coconut Oil
Ghee (Clarified Butter)
Macadamia Nut Oil
Olive Oil
Sunflower Oil
Safflower Oil

Nuts and Seeds
Almonds **
Brazil Nuts**
Cashews**
Chia Seeds**
Hazelnuts**
Hemp Seeds**
Macadamias**
Pecans**
Pine Nuts**
Pistachios**
Pumpkin Seeds**
Sesame Seeds**
Sunflower Seeds**
Walnuts**

Spices [ALL spices]
Allspice

Anise
Basil
Bay Leaf
Black Pepper
Cardamom
Cayenne Pepper
Celery Seed
Chili Pepper
Chili Powder
Cilantro
Cinnamon
Cloves
Coriander Seeds
Cumin
Curry-Green
Curry-Red
Curry-Yellow
Dill
Fennel
Fenugreek
Garam Masala
Garlic
Ginger
Herbs de Provence
Mint
Mustard Seeds
Nutmeg
Oregano
Paprika
Peppermint
Rosemary
Sage
Salt

Tarragon
Thyme
Turmeric

Dairy
Butter
Ghee
Fermented Yogurt*
Greek Yogurt*
Kefir*
Heavy Whipping
Cream

Fruits [Low GL]
Lime (1 GL)
Strawberry (1 GL)
Fresh Apricot (3 GL)
Fresh Cherries (3 GL)
Grapefruit (3 GL)
Lemon (3 GL)
Watermelon (4 GL)
Cantaloupe (4 GL)
Guava (4 GL)
Nectarines (4 GL)
Oranges (4 GL)
Pear (4 GL)
Watermelon (4 GL)
Fresh Blueberries (5 GL)
Fresh Peaches (5 GL)
Fresh Plums (5 GL)

Other
Beef Broth

Nut Butters	Lime Juice	Vinegar
Chicken Broth	Mustard	
Coconut Milk	Pesto	**Sweeteners**
Fish Sauce	Salsa	Erythritol
Hot Sauce	Soy Sauce	Monk Fruit
Hummus	Sriracha	Stevia
Lemon Juice	Tamari (wheat free)	

* These foods are high in net carbohydrates and should only be consumed after you have reached your goal weight. They're not to be consumed if your goal is fat loss.

** These foods are technically okay but are very easy to overdo. They should be limited to small snacks only.

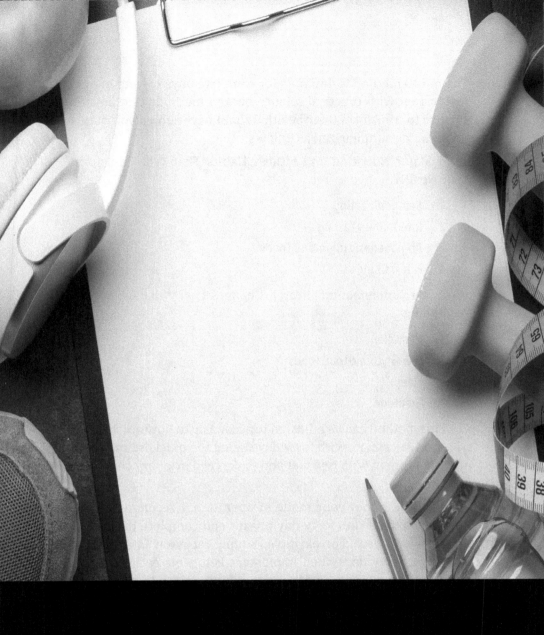

Summary

The mR40 method is designed for complete physical and mental restoration with practical science-backed methods that anyone can use to transform their health. What I have shown you in this book can be summarized as follows:

4 Major Nutrition and Fitness Habits That Will Transform Your Health

1. Ketogenic Eating
2. Intermittent Fasting
3. Angiogenesis-Inhibiting Foods
4. HIIT Training

And 4 Supplemental Lifestyle Changes That Will Elevate Your Well-being

1. Hydration
2. Low-Glycemic-Load Foods
3. Sleep
4. Gratitude

This method can be adjusted to according to how quickly you want to see change, with forty days being the quickest and most intense. Jump in with two feet and make revolutionary change in your life.

If "all in" is not your mode of operation, I recommend you break each habit into forty-day phases and complete them over the span of a year. For example: Simply focus on intermittent fasting for forty days, then implement ketogenic eating for the next forty days, then angiogenesis-inhibiting foods, then HIIT training, and so forth and so on. During each phase you will put your main focus on that one habit. Not that you won't attempt to sleep well or hydrate but rather most of your effort will go toward your main goal. In less than a year you will have transformed your lifestyle and your health.

Please share your results on social media using the hashtag #mR40methodResults. I am so excited to see and hear your results.

Committed to your success,

Mubarakah Ibrahim

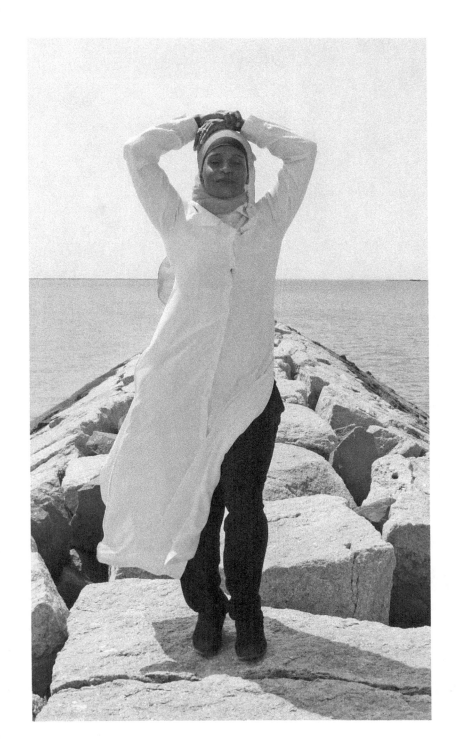

CPSIA information can be obtained
at www.ICGtesting.com
Printed in the USA
FSHW022118120120
65790FS